Traditional Taekwondo

Traditional Taekwondo

Core Techniques, History, and Philosophy

Doug Cook

YMAA Publication Center
Boston, Mass. USA

YMAA Publication Center, Inc.
Main Office
4354 Washington Street
Boston, Massachusetts, 02131
1-800-669-8892 • www.ymaa.com • ymaa@aol.com

Editor: Susan Bullowa
Cover Design: Richard Rossiter

ISBN-10: 1-59439-066-5
ISBN-13: 978-1-59439-066-1

10   9   8   7   6   5   4   3   2   1

Publisher's Cataloging in Publication

Cook, Doug.

Traditional taekwondo : core techniques, history, and philosophy /
Doug Cook. -- Boston, Mass. : YMAA Publication Center, 2006.

p. ; cm.
ISBN-13: 978-1-59439-066-1
ISBN-10: 1-59439-066-5
Includes bibliographical references and index.

1. Tae kwon do.
I. Title.

GV1114.9 .C66 2006   2006922723
796.815/3--dc22   0604

Disclaimer:
The author and publisher of this material are NOT RESPONSIBLE in any manner whatsoever for
any injury which may occur through reading or following the instructions in this manual.
The activities, physical or otherwise, described in this material may be too strenuous or dangerous
for some people, and the reader(s) should consult a physician before engaging in them.

The author wishes to assure the reader that the use of the personal pronouns "he or "she" do not imply
the exclusion of any person.

In an effort to avoid confusion, the author has chosen to conform to the western custom of placing
surnames last rather than first which is routine in Asia. The only exception is General Choi, Hong Hi
since he is universally recognized by this iteration.

Printed in Canada.

Table of Contents

This book is dedicated to My Father and Mother,
Roy Lee Douglas Cook and Joan Millicent Ashcroft Cook,
for preparing me from birth with love and encouragement,
for my journey along The Way. To whatever Energy governs us,

Bless Them.

Foreword

Over the centuries, it has become a tradition in the martial arts for students to carry forth the teachings of their master instructors from generation to generation. Although much has changed, partially due to the advent of combat sport coupled with the modern school owner's pursuit of commercial success at any cost, this custom continues unabated in all classical disciplines. Therefore, it is with great pleasure that I observe one of my own students perpetuating this principle by faithfully transmitting traditional taekwondo technique both physically and academically with forethought, integrity, and vision. Clearly, Master Doug Cook, the author of this work, has chosen to take the road less traveled; a path that requires courage since it places high demands on the students who train under him.

More than ever, martial arts schools abound that have forfeited ritual practice in favor of classes that feature aerobic-oriented exercise along with a hodgepodge of technique borrowed from various cultures. Contrary to this approach, Master Cook and his school, the Chosun Taekwondo Academy, continues to provide a pure and authentic form of taekwondo within the bounds of a curriculum rich in self-defense, forms, philosophy, meditation, and internal energy, or *Ki*, development exercises that holistically stimulate the mind, body, and spirit. I am deeply gratified to see that he has chosen this course since it dovetails perfectly with my personal method of instruction thus satisfying the time-honored tradition of succession.

Aside from the attention given to the physical and spiritual components of traditional taekwondo, Doug Cook, following in my footsteps, contributes academically to the martial arts community at large through his command of the written word. His previously published book titled *Taekwondo: Ancient Wisdom for the Modern Warrior* has become a standard in schools and universities across the nation and around the world. In this, his second book, he juxtaposes the philosophical content of his first work against the historical and technical information contained here. In the pages that follow, the reader will discover a section concentrating on the history of Korea, the homeland of taekwondo, which will add color and texture to their training. Moreover, the author offers a vivid description of the organizations and personalities that played a major role in the evolution of taekwondo during its formative years; a subject few have tackled since accurate information is so scarce. *Poom-Se*, the formal exercises that represent the essence of taekwondo, meditation, and *Ki* development exercises, too, are given the much-deserved editorial space they deserve. Then, adding to the historical and metaphysical aspects of the martial arts, this exciting work also depicts many practical self-defense strategies that escalate in complexity and subsequently will prove beneficial to the novice and advanced black-belt holder alike. Taken in total, the two volumes comprise a body of knowledge essential to a comprehensive understanding of traditional taekwondo. With this in mind, I wholeheartedly recommend this book to all taekwondo practitioners and to those practicing related disciplines who wish to elevate their knowledge of self-defense, philosophy, and the history and culture of the traditional Korean martial art of taekwondo.

Grandmaster Richard Chun
9th Dan Black Belt
President
United States Taekwondo Association

Acknowledgements

As with any literary venture, there are people, places and objects that directly or indirectly influence the direction of the work. Subsequently, I would like to thank, demonstrate my appreciation to, and make mention of the following:

Grandmaster Richard Chun for his tireless efforts in promoting traditional taekwondo and for initially accepting me as a student; Master Samuel Mizrahi for his patience and for being an exemplary training partner…you are my inspiration; Master Pablo Alejandro for his knowledge and technical skill; My soon-to-be-ancient Dell Inspiron 4100; David Ripianzi of YMAA for his integrity, vision and promises kept; Katy Glover and the Albert Wisner Public Library, Warwick, NY; The instructors and students of the Chosun Taekwondo Academy; My editor Susan Bullowa for pulling it all together; Tim Comrie and John Jordon III for their photographic skills; Carol Davis Hart of Tae Kwon Do Times magazine; Sung Kyung Kim of the Korean National Tourism Organization for her help in providing outstanding graphics and research; The virtue of Perseverance; Michael and John Lee of Honda Martial Arts Supply, NYC; The Grandmasters and Masters of the past who dedicated their lives to the martial arts; As always, Starbucks; Patricia Lurye and Christine Indorato for their dedication to the Chosun Taekwondo Academy and for their assistance in data entry; Denny, David and Dawn; My Muse for its generosity and for filling me with the proper words.

But most of all…Patricia Ann, Erin Elizabeth, and Kristin Lee Cook, the breath of my life, for the love, support, and encouragement they give that I can only hope to return in equal measure.

Special thanks go to my students, Cheryl Crouchen, Peter Brawley, Dr. Andrew Hirsch, Daniel Lane, and Patricia Cook for participating in the technical sequences demonstrated in this book. Your exemplary skill, patience, and contribution to the art of traditional taekwondo is deeply appreciated.

MEMBER:
THE UNITED STATES TAEKWONDO ASS'N.
THE WORLD TAEKWONDO FEDERATION

220 EAST 86TH STREET
NEW YORK, N.Y. 10028
TEL: (212) 772-3700

Richard Chun Taekwondo Center, Inc.

Dear Sabum Doug Cook,

It is with great delight that I write this letter of recommendation to celebrate the publication of your latest work, <u>Traditional Taekwondo—Core Techniques, History, and Philosophy</u>, by YMAA Publication Center of Boston. In view of the success of your first book, I am certain that martial artists worldwide, regardless of style, will benefit greatly from your supreme effort.

Clearly, the teaching of taekwondo in a traditional manner is currently at a premium, yet in your writing, you support it with pride. This is a joy to see and a relief knowing that which I have devoted my life to will be carried forward with dignity by one of my senior students.

It is worth mentioning that my colleagues, high-ranking masters all, have taken notice of your accomplishments, often commenting to me that you have become a recognized authority on the history and philosophy of the Korean national martial art of taekwondo. Therefore, please accept this correspondence with my congratulations and the heart felt gratitude of the taekwondo community at large. On behalf of the United States Taekwondo Association, I wish you and your taekwondo center good fortune now and in the future.

Sincerely yours,

Grand Master Richard Chun
9th dan black belt
President
USTA

Preface

Defining Traditional Taekwondo

Taekwondo, literally translated, can be defined as "foot, hand, Way" or "the Way of smashing with hands and feet." Such descriptive nomenclature understandably implies a curriculum rich in self-defense. Too often, however, this is simply not the case. Given the current popularity of sports competition in the martial arts, many techniques of defensive value have been stripped away or forfeited altogether in favor of those certain to score in the ring. While the thirst for Olympic gold has clearly played a significant role in propelling taekwondo into the forefront, it should be remembered that the native Korean martial art contains over 3200 distinct techniques. These include a multitude of blocks, kicks, and strikes, in addition to a variety of leg sweeps, joint locks, and throws, truly qualifying it as a complete form of self-defense.

Consequently, in an effort to preserve the formal nature and defensive infrastructure of taekwondo as originally intended by a portion of its founders, a number of training institutes or *dojangs* now promote what is referred to as *traditional taekwondo;* an alternative style emphasizing a core philosophy rich in basic technique, *poom-se,* and authentic defensive strategy with little or no emphasis on competition, thus divorcing it somewhat from its sports-oriented mate.

Nevertheless, this classification may be construed as somewhat of a misnomer since, as we shall see, the history or "tradition" of taekwondo, as it exists today, is relatively short with much of it being devoted to its promotion as a world sport. Like it or not, the answer to this paradox lays in the fact that taekwondo owes much of its pedigree to foreign influences, some of which are rooted in Funikoshi's

태권도

Taekwondo: "Foot, Hand, Way" in Hangul.

Shotokan karate-do, Ushiba's aikido, Kano's Kodokan judo, and to a lesser degree, Chinese gungfu. This is no accident given the geopolitical climate that existed in Korea during the turbulent years of the early to mid 1900s. In fact, to the experienced eye, many of the martial applications illustrated in this book, having been handed down over the decades if not centuries, bear a striking resemblance to those fashioned by the founders listed above. Subsequently, in its evolutionary stage, prior to its promotion as an Olympic sport, taekwondo contained a complete palette of defensive techniques. With this in mind, the notion of taekwondo having a "traditional" component based on strong basic skills, forms or *poom-se*, and self-defense, predating the creation of organizations promoting its sports-oriented component, materializes.

Although this work will focus mainly on the defensive tactics of traditional taekwondo and the training elements that support them, it should be understood that these alone do not satisfy the conditions necessary to formalize taekwondo as a traditional martial art. As stated above, the practice of forms, coupled with the fundamentals and the philosophical underpinnings that comprise them, lay at the core of any traditional martial discipline. In recognition of this fact, traditional taekwondo *poom-se* training represents the essence of the art and is a direct reflection of its unique character and heritage. While it is true that many of the forms practiced by the taekwondoist mirror those of rival Asian martial arts, it only goes to prove that in the past diverse martial disciplines from the region drew from a common well in an effort to construct practical, combat proven formal exercises. Despite the fact that these exercises by now have largely been Korean-ized, they embody universal defensive movements that date back to antiquity further supporting the traditional nature of taekwondo.

Moreover, a traditional martial art should embrace an overriding philosophy governed by a set or moral principles that limit its use to situations of grave necessity. In addition, this philosophical doctrine, while enhancing the character of the martial artist, should reflect the cultural values extant in the discipline's nation of origin. In the case of traditional taekwondo, these ethical guidelines date back to the seventh century when warriors of the Hwarang, an elite corps of young nobles, sought guidance from the Buddhist monk Wonkwang Popsa before entering battle. This moral compass, as we shall see, continues to be followed to this day by the practitioner of traditional taekwondo.

A Proven Combat Art

Yet, according to Kane and Wilder, even further evidence is required for a martial art to be branded *traditional*. In their book, *The Way of Kata*, the authors state that, "traditional study of martial systems presumes the ability to perform techniques in actual combat. Sport and conditioning applications are more or less fringe benefits associated with such study." Using this condition as a yardstick to further measure the traditional value of taekwondo, we must establish that a militaristic legacy exists using the available evidence at hand.

History demonstrates that for centuries Korean warriors have stood ready to defend their nation at a moments notice. Rarely, until today, have we in the west experienced such necessity for vigilance. While much of this warfare involved the use of bows, arrows, swords and firearms, there have been many occasions where empty-hand self-defense tactics contributed to victory. In 1592, fighting monks, keepers of martial arts skills that had all but vanished during the pro-Confucian Yi Dynasty, were recruited in an effort to resist a massive Japanese force lead by Toyotomi Hideyoshi intent on using the Korean peninsula as a stepping stone to China. Later, in the years following the conclusion of World War II and the Japanese Occupation, government officials approached Won Kuk Lee, founder of the Chung Do Kwan, requesting that he enlist the help of his students in quelling the civil disobedience created by roving bands of desperate citizens.

In 1953, another milestone was planted solidifying taekwondo as a legitimate form of self-defense when General Choi, Hong Hi created the 29th Infantry Division at the request of General Sun Yub Baek, chief of staff of the Korean Army. Symbolized by an insignia depicting a fist over the Korean peninsula, the "fist" or Il Keu Division distinguished itself by marrying regulation drills with martial arts training, marking it as a truly unique entity within the Korean military.

But the great wheel of progress in the development of a unified Korean martial art with a complete defensive strategy did not stop there. In 1962 perhaps one of the most significant events in validating taekwondo as an effective combat art occurred. President Go Din Diem of South Vietnam requested that the Korean government send representatives of their native martial art to instruct the Vietnamese military in taekwondo.

This initial group was lead by Major Tae Hee Nam of the Oh Do Kwan. As the war escalated, however, the number of instructors ultimately grew to 647. In an article published shortly before his death, General Choi stated that "The strength of taekwondo training in Korean soldiers had a psychological effect on the Viet Cong." In fact, this training became so effective that the Viet Cong directed their troops to retreat rather then confront the taekwondo-trained soldiers. Even today, the black-uniformed White Tigers, a group within the elite Korean Army Black Beret unit, practices a new form of empty-hand combat art known as *tuck kong moo sool*.

Moreover, the Korean Army is not the only beneficiary of taekwondo martial applications. U. S. Army troops stationed in Korea have traditionally been exposed to native martial arts. Even today, American armed forces of the Army's 2nd Infantry Division have adopted taekwondo, in conjunction with jujutsu, as their primary form of martial arts practice. Nicknamed, the Warrior Division, 14,000 soldiers celebrate the sun-rise each day with a series of Korean self-defense tactics. Using *kihops* as their battle cry, these modern day warriors are not interested in merely sparring for the sport of it, but seek to increase confidence, perhaps the single most important ingredient of survival on the battlefield, through the development of traditional taekwondo self-defense skills. Additional goals of the program include improving physical fitness, cultivating disciplined teamwork through the practice of the classical forms, and gaining a better understanding of Korea's rich cultural heritage. Just as in any civilian *dojang*, military personnel drill in the kicks, strikes, blocks, throws, and sweeps that lie at the core of traditional taekwondo. Implemented in January 2001, Warrior Taekwondo, as it has come to be called, is a resounding success with plans to expand the program to include all U.S. forces in Korea.

Contrary to the historical evidence at hand, critics who support the perception that taekwondo has evolved into nothing more then a popular combat sport continue to debate the fundamental defensive value of the art. Further compounding this issue, it is

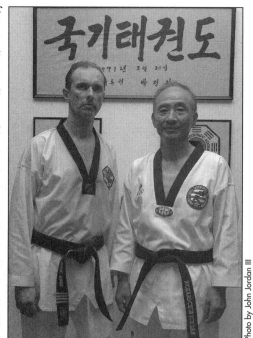

Grandmaster Richard Chun (right) with Master Doug Cook.

becoming increasingly difficult to locate an instructor faithful to the principles unique to traditional taekwondo. This dilemma is made all the more poignant in an article published by the late writer and martial arts instructor Jane Hallender titled, *Is Taekwondo a Sport or a Self-defense System?* Acutely aware of the differences, Hallender warns, "There is more to taekwondo than just tournament competition. From kicks, to hand strikes, to throws, to joint locks, taekwondo possesses an array of defensive measures designed to thwart virtually any kind of attack. The most difficult part will not be learning the self-defense techniques, but finding a taekwondo instructor who still teaches them."

Preserving Tradition

In spite of this, practitioners true to the defensive nature of taekwondo do exist; it is simply a matter of seeking them out. One prime example of an instructor possessing these skills is martial arts pioneer Grandmaster Richard Chun, 9th Dan and president of the United States Taekwondo Association (USTA), an organization whose mission is to "promote excellence in an ancient and evolving art". Assigning

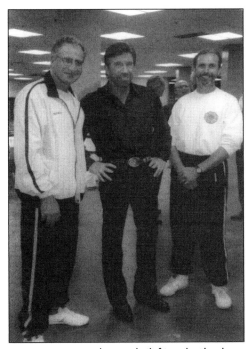

Master Samuel Mizrah (left) with Chuck Norris and Master Cook during a demonstration at Madison Square Garden, New York.

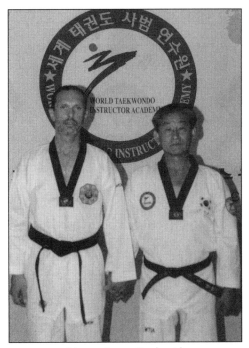

Master Doug Cook with Grandmaster Gyoo Hyun Lee (right).

great attention to self-defense tactics, forms, and basic skills, Grandmaster Chun, in conjunction with his senior instructors Samuel Mizrahi and Pablo Alejandro, teach students that taekwondo is not merely a sport, but a way of life, a form of protection, and a path to self-fulfillment.

However, the list of instructors who have immigrated to America with the express purpose of advancing the traditional martial art of taekwondo does not stop there. Outstanding teachers such as Grandmaster Jhoon Rhee, Byung Min Kim, Yeon Hee Park, Daeshik Kim, Sijak Henry Cho, and Seon Duk Son have also contributed greatly to the refinement of Korean defensive strategy. But, in order to sample and appreciate the true flavor of traditional taekwondo self-defense tactics, it is sometimes necessary to visit their country of origin.

In the summer of 1995, 1999, and again in 2004, my school, the Chosun Taekwondo Academy, had the honor of accompanying Grandmaster Richard Chun and a group of other USTA members on a training and cultural tour of Korea. Aside from appreciating the rich, native heritage of the Korean people, we were given an

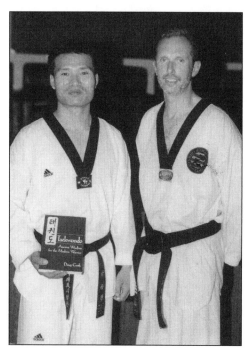

Master Doug Cook with Grandmaster
Seung Hyeon Nam (right).

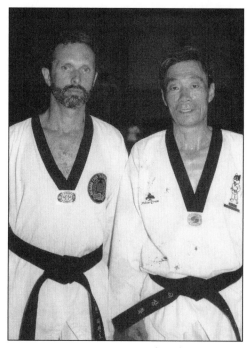

Master Doug Cook with
Grandmaster Sang Hak Lee.

opportunity to train with some of the most noted instructors in the world. One such professional, apart from Grandmasters Gyoo Hyun Lee, founder of the World Taekwondo Instructor Academy and Seung Hyeon Nam of Kyung Won University, was Grandmaster Sang Hak Lee who was responsible for training the Korean Army Ranger Corps and National Police Agency in self-defense, and was head of a select team of martial artists sent to Vietnam to demonstrate the practicality of taekwondo.

In his instructional methodology, Grandmaster Lee, a tall trim gentleman with a ruddy complexion, moved effortlessly through the various traditional martial applications he chose to gift us with. In demonstration, he allowed his opponent's aggressive behavior to betray him through the redirection of punches, kicks, and grabs, thus manifesting the true defensive philosophy of traditional taekwondo. He did not speak much, choosing instead to perform each technique with the spirit one comes to expect from an experienced, Korean master. By the end of the afternoon, somewhat bruised and overwhelmed, we were given over twenty self-defense tactics to take home to America. Some of these appear here along side those of his aforementioned counterparts who continue their practice in this country.

Aside from providing the practitioner with a brief glimpse into the historical tradition, theory and philosophy of traditional taekwondo, coupled with the defensive strategy it supports, it is my intention to share these skills in detail with the reader using the technical section of this book as a guide.

Finally, the practice of traditional taekwondo is a highly fulfilling experience. If approached with sincerity, the rewards are great, physically, mentally and spiritually. However, I respectfully hope that martial artists of all disciplines will benefit from this work.

PART ONE

History and Culture

CHAPTER 1

Introduction

Korea is a nation that is no stranger to life's struggle for survival. Since the days of the Hwarang in the seventh century to the bloody civil conflict between the North and South in the 1950s, its warriors have been pressed into battle in an effort to preserve the sovereignty of the strategically significant peninsula. A stretch of landmass about the size of Indiana jutting down into the Yellow Sea, its defenses have been breached hundreds of times over the centuries by invading forces using its proximity as a stepping stone to the vastness of China. A visit to Korea today, however, reveals little in the way of its embattled past. One cannot help but admire the lush rolling hills and terraced rice paddies that dot the countryside. Inhabitants of Seoul, its capitol city, stroll or ride bicycles along wide, common areas lining the Han River. The Namdaemun marketplace is awash in a sea of humanity where the buyer can purchase anything from authentic celadon vases to strips of dried squid. Traffic snarls its narrow streets and everywhere ornate temples are in evidence, confirming a deepseated belief in Buddhist and Confucian ethics. A thriving industrial complex, in tandem with a juxtaposition of modern and traditional architecture, stands in proud testimony to a humble yet tenacious citizenry.

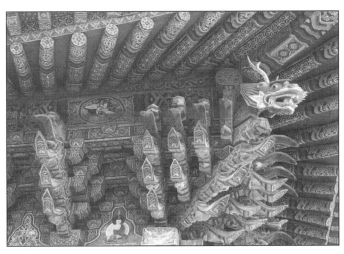

Temple Roof Carvings.

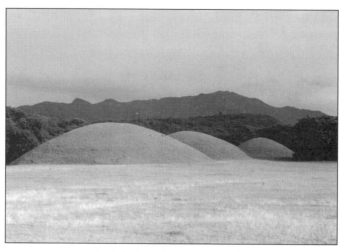

Burial Mounds at Tumuli Park.

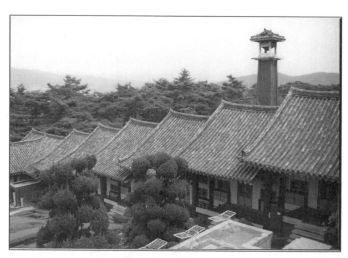

The Hwarang Training Institute.

In 1961, national security advisor W.W. Rostow argued in favor of this tenacity in a memo titled "Action in Korea" prepared for then president, John F. Kennedy. In the memo, Rostow recognized Korea's people as its greatest resource. This spirit for survival, the raw will to persevere regardless of what, to many, would have appeared insurmountable odds, represents the foundation and philosophical backbone of traditional taekwondo self-defense doctrine.

In order to gain a better understanding of the circumstances and personalities surrounding the creation of this highly effective Asian martial art, literally translated as "foot, hand, Way" or "the Way of smashing with hands and feet," it is important that we take a moment to view its legacy through the window of Korean history. Revisiting this historical mosaic will only serve to amplify a past that has cultivated an environment where self-defense, both in a practical and emotional sense, became essential. Why take the time to familiarize the martial artist with an overview of Korean history and not simply technique? Just as the geography of a region influences the physical aspects of a given martial art, so the mold of history shapes its philosophical and spiritual component. Let us begin our explorations at the dawn of Asian culture, and then progress to a time when, out of necessity, the indigenous martial arts of ancient Korea were held in high regard and a confederation of states were first beginning to taste the fruits of unification.

CHAPTER 2
Historical Periods

KO-CHOSUN (2333 BC): LAND OF THE MORNING CALM

Before the warriors of the Hwarang and the Sunbae appeared, before the battles for unification of the Korean peninsula were fought and won, it is said that in the year 2333 BC, Hwanung, son of the divine being Hwanin, descended from heaven to the top of Mount Baekdoo with express instructions to create a new country in the eastern lands. Not far away in a small cave dwelt a bear and a tiger, each of whom in their own way desired to become human. Upon overhearing the prayers of the bear and tiger, Hwanung offered to grant their wish under the condition that they remain secluded in a cave for one hundred days, eating nothing but the garlic cloves and artemisia that he provided. Because of the tiger's innate restlessness, he was unable to meet this demand. The bear, on the other hand whose patience prevailed, exited the cave as a beautiful maiden and was given the name Ungyo. Hwanung was so taken with Ungyo's magnificence that he requested her to become his bride. Miraculously, following the transmission on Hwanung's breath of life, she gave birth to a son, naming him Tan-gun. After uniting the six northern tribes, Tan-gun, considered the progenitor of present-day Korea, established the nation, Ko-Chosun, or "Land of the Morning Calm."

Raised by the ancients, Tan-gun went on to help civilize the uncultivated tribes by teaching them farming, architecture, and various social graces. More importantly, however, the mythical founder is credited with originating a traditional, national philosophy through his advocacy of *hongik-ingan* (the benefits of universal humanism) and *jaese-ihwa* (the rationalization of human living). These concepts, especially *hongik-ingan*, which codifies the Korean sense of duty to the state, family, and forebearers, constitute the foundation of a social framework that has blossomed into the uniquely Korean culture that exists today. Furthermore, the ancients needed to reconcile the ruthlessness of the elements, natural phenomenon, and a highly restrictive lifestyle by clinging to a belief in "heaven's god," or impeccable virtuousness, later known as seon. According to the *Taekwon-Do Textbook*, published under the auspices of the Kukkiwon in Seoul, Korea, these doctrines have done much in contributing to

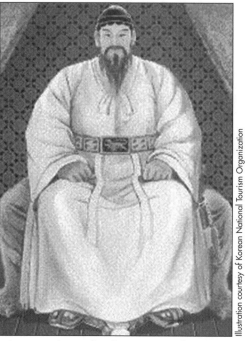

Illustration courtesy of Korean National Tourism Organization

Tan-gun, the mythical progenitor of Korea.

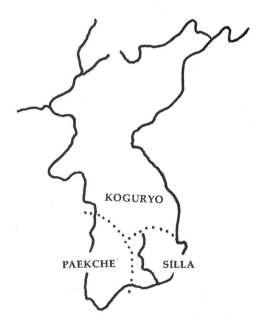

KOGURYO

PAEKCHE   SILLA

Map of the Three Kingdoms.

the *Do*, or the Way, of taekwondo as well as the overall character of traditional and contemporary Korean ethics.

THE THREE KINGDOMS AND UNITED SILLA PERIOD (57 BCE–935 AD)

Two thousand years ago, the Korean peninsula was divided into three discreet kingdoms called Silla (57 BCE–935 AD), Koguryo (37 BCE–668 AD), and Paekche (18 BCE–660 CE). These territories, composed of tribes overseen by powerful warlords, were constantly at war in an attempt to expand their territorial reach, and riddled by internal strife. Because there was a genuine fear of invasion by neighboring countries such as Japan, skilled warriors and the military class were held in high regard. As a result, Koguryo, the largest of the three kingdoms with land holdings reaching far up into what is now North Korea and Manchuria, established a warrior corps that came to be known as the Sunbae. Essentially meaning "senior," Sunbae philosophy was underscored by a deep belief in the gods who created the universe coupled with a strong will to defend the country against all odds. These philosopher/warriors, selected from all rungs of society, wore black velvet clothing and shaved their heads. The Sunbae were democratic in nature in that anyone, given high aptitude and an ambitious character, could obtain superior rank.

8

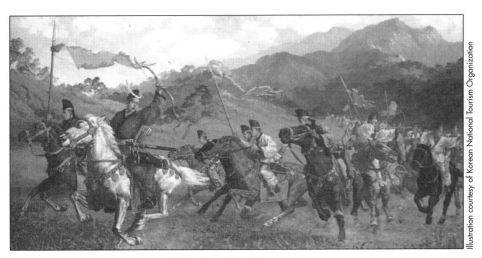

Illustration courtesy of Korean National Tourism Organization

Warriors of the Hwarang.

Likewise, in 37 AD, Silla, the smallest of the three kingdoms, established a military fraternity under the direction of King Jin Heung, patterned after the Sunbae troops, but christened the Hwarang. Unlike the Sunbae, however, members of the Hwarang, practicing Hwarang-do or the "Way of the Flowering Manhood," were comprised of elite warriors exclusively drawn from noble stock. Aside from their knowledge of *kwonbop* and *subak*, two native martial arts of the day, these youthful soldiers were distinguished from other combat troops by virtue of their unique holistic training in archery, music, poetry, equestrian skills, and the Eastern philosophical paradigms of Confucianism, Buddhism and Taoism.

Moreover, the Hwarang lived under a strict code of honor handed down by the Buddhist monk, Wonkwang Popsa. These basic moral principles, included loyalty to the king, filial piety and restraint against misuse of force in battle. When not engaged in battle, Hwarang warriors were known to train in the mountains, provide support to those experiencing difficult times, and make repairs to roads and castles.

In 668, with the aid of China who often assumed the protective role of big brother in coming to the aid of its smaller sibling, the Sillian leadership, using the Hwarang as their instrument of war, succeeded in bringing the three kingdoms under central control. Subsequently, historians mark this date as the beginning of a unified Korea under the banner of United Silla.

For more then 230 years, the region enjoyed peace and prosperity. Culturally, with Buddhism and Confucianism quickly becoming the predominant philosophies, magnificent temples were constructed throughout the land. Built during the reign of King Pophung (reigned 514-540), Bulguksa Temple located in Kyongju, remains today one of the most striking and is considered a magnificent example of Sillian architecture.

However, as taught by Taoist doctrine, change is inevitable and even United Silla was not immune to this universal dynamic. Social discontent, high taxation and decadence among its rulers began to replace the accomplishments of the past, effectively ending this golden age in Korean history.

THE KORYO DYNASTY (918–1392 AD)

The 475 years following the United Silla era represented a period of growth and reorganization. Thirty-seven kings ruled over wondrous advances that became the hallmark of the Koryo Dynasty. In 1234, moveable metal type was invented, preceding Guttenberg by 200 years. Celadon porcelain, developed by Koryo artisans and noted for its colorful glaze, to this day captures the attention of collectors. Perhaps one of the

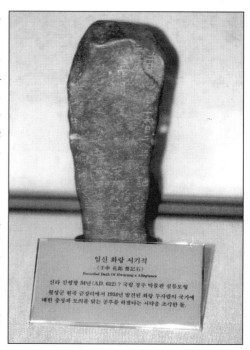

Stone tablet inscribed with ethical guidelines practiced by the Hwarang.

greatest legacies of this time was the publication of the *Tripitaka Koreana*, or Buddhist sutras. Believing that the power of prayer would turn back the Mongol invasion, Buddhist monks undertook the task of engraving over 80,000 wooden plates containing the most sacred of scriptures. Requiring 16 years to complete, the *Tripitaka* now resides in the safety of Haeinsa Temple.

Korean Buddhism embraced a martial component as well in the form of the Subdue Demon Corps who are credited with holding off the Jurchen invaders. Fighting monks bearing martial arts skills were not uncommon during this period. This fact is particularly evident given the techniques taught by the Zen patriarch Bodhidharma at the Shaolin Temple located in China's Hunan Province. Forbidden to use weapons of any kind, these monks relied on the fighting arts to protect themselves from roving bandits and as a defense against wild animals on their travels throughout the countryside. As a religious paradigm, however, Buddhism began to wane in favor of the more practical teachings of Confucius.

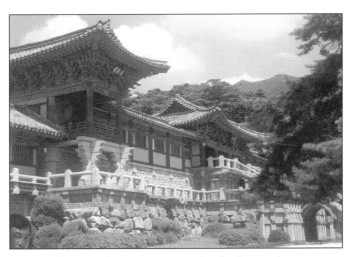

Bulguksa Temple, a prime example of Sillian architecture.

THE YI (CHOSUN) DYNASTY (1392–1910 AD)

The Yi, or Chosun Dynasty , last of the great dynastic successions, gave rise to many noted leaders and military tacticians not the least being its founding ruler and namesake, General Song Gye Yi. By this time, the virtuous effects of Buddhism had spun out of control poisoning the upper echelons of Koryo government. Leaders were required to become Buddhist monks as a prerequisite to kingship. The last of the Koryo monarchs, against the will of the people and ignoring the fact that China had proven itself a worthy ally for so long, ordered Yi to mount an attack against Ming forces garrisoned in Manchuria. General Yi, with the unanimous support of the general populace, refused, laying siege to the capitol instead. This resulted in the ousting of the unpopular Koryo ruler and the installation of Song Gye Yi as the first Chosun monarch. As a backlash to the abuses of the Buddhist priesthood, Confucianism became the dominant philosophy allowing civilians rather then the clergy to fill the halls of power.

The practice of native martial arts faded somewhat into the background during the Yi Dynasty in no small part due to the introduction of gunpowder and other technological advances on the battlefield. These innovations, however, did not erase the indomitable will of one remarkable Korean warrior and admiral whom we shall meet shortly.

Japan, unlike China, had proven to be a viable threat as far back as the Three Kingdoms period when pirates originating from the island nation would constantly make incursions into Sillian territory. Consequently, in May of 1592, Toyotomi Hideyoshi, a powerful warlord who had successfully united contentious military groups within his country, lead a fleet of ships carrying 158,700 soldiers in an assault on the Korean peninsula; this in response to the Chosun leadership's refusal for aid in attacking China. Sadly, two centuries of quietude had taken its toll greatly diminishing the nation's ability to defend itself. After making landfall in the south near Pusan, Hideyoshi's troops, armed with superior firepower, defiantly swept north meeting little resistance along the way.

Then, with the future of Chosun literally hanging in the balance, a hero arose as if by divine intervention in the shape of Admiral Sun Shin Yi.

Admiral Yi, by all standards, was a brilliant naval strategist best known for his invention of the *kobukson*, or turtle boat that was the first ironclad ship ever to rule the seas. Constructed by engineer Na Tae Yong to Yi's specifications, the vessel measured 65 feet long and 15 feet amidships with a topmast reaching 90 feet in height.

Fire arrows and sulfur-laden smoke issued forth from four cannons positioned in the mouth of a carved turtle head mounted on its bow. Sharpened

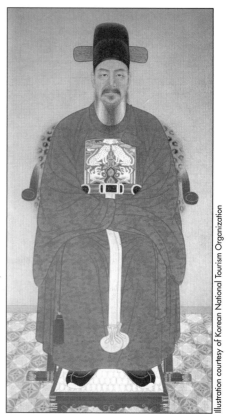

Admiral Sun Shin Yi.

Illustration courtesy of Korean National Tourism Organization

spears protruded from the deck with all vital areas covered by armor. The sight of a *kobukson* appearing over the horizon was certain to strike fear in the hearts of the enemy. Over the course of the next seven years, Sun Shin Yi's fleet of turtle boats would dominate the waters off Korea. Three times, he would decimate the Japanese navy with unique military maneuvers such as the "fishnet" never before seen in battle. Finally, in 1598, after galvanizing local guerrilla units to defend against enemy land forces, Yi would ultimately claim victory over the Japanese, but not before forfeiting his own life in the line of duty.

Military might and political intrigue notwithstanding, the brightest jewel in the crown of cultural achievement was set by one of the most revered leaders in Korean history. The fifth son of Yi Song Gwe, King Sejong (reigned 1418-1450) was responsible for the invention of *hangul*, the unique Korean alphabet consisting of 24 letters and lauded by linguists for its accuracy in phonetically representing the sounds of native words.

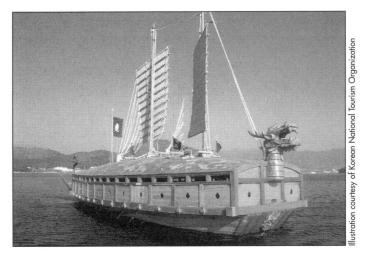

Kobukson, or turtle boat.

Referred to originally as *hunmin chongum*, or "proper sounds to instruct the people," this most recent of global alphabets was intended by its originator to do just that. Until then, Chinese with its extensive system of pictographs had been the method of choice used by academics in expressing the written word. The adoption of *hangul* permitted the average citizen to access literature and communicate with one another through writing.

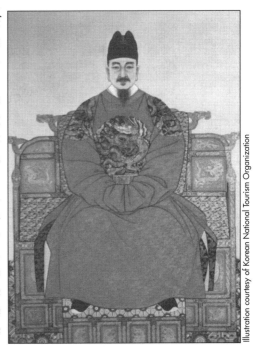

Known as the Leonardo da Vinci of the region for his talents and innovation, King Sejong was also involved in the development of timepieces, moveable metal type, and a 365-volume medical encyclopedia.

The years following Admiral Sun Shin Yi's defeat of the Japanese navy saw Korea withdrawing even more into itself with a distinct trend towards isolationism. Japan, meanwhile, was fueling its soon-to-be monolithic engine of industry while the Chosun King Yongjo was confounded by the perplexities of his pathological son, Prince Sado. Until the latter part of the eighteenth

King Sejong.

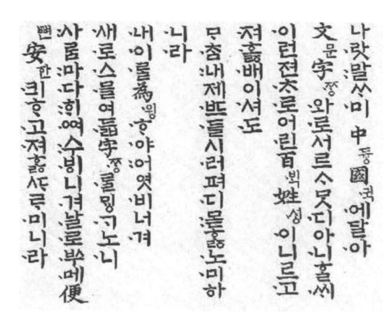

Hangul, the Korean alphabet created by King Sejong in 1443.

century, the Korean people, with their nation being dubbed "The Hermit Kingdom," were largely unaware of the comings and goings of the Western world, thinking that instead the seat of civilization was centered in India or China. This narrow world view was about to be inextricably altered with the advent of Catholicism, rumors of technological advances heralded by traveling envoys, new bloodlines introduced by ship-wrecked sailors, and the political manipulations of the major world powers who were guilty of ignoring the cries of a nation that was about to be set upon by the humiliation of colonialism.

THE JAPANESE OCCUPATION (1910 – 1945 AD)

With Russia's advance into Manchuria during the 1890s, Japan's imperialistic gaze again fell on Korea fearing further expansion by the Russian military. In 1898, a noninterference agreement was signed by representatives of both weary governments that profoundly affected the fate of Korea. Still, this agreement did not preclude the eventual outbreak of war in 1904 between the two nations. In spite of Korea's proclamation of neutrality, Japan began to openly infiltrate its government by sending advisors to oversee the operations of its various branches. Japan surprised the world the following year by claiming victory over Russia, thus putting an end to the Russo-Japanese war. By signing the Treaty of Portsmouth, however, Russia essentially gave the green light to the eradication of Korea's right to self-rule.

For years, Japan had been negotiating with foreign powers in brokering approval to colonize its neighbor. Finally on August 22, 1910, Japan officially annexed the Korean peninsula effectively bringing an end to 519 years of continuous leadership under the Chosun Dynasty. For all intents and purposes, the final nail had been hammered into the coffin of Korean independence. While some posit that the imperial Japanese contributed to the Korean infrastructure through the construction of railways, roads and communication systems, there is little doubt that any convenience created was disproportionately offset by the pain and suffering perpetrated on the Korean populace as a whole. In 1910 alone, over 300,000 books were publicly burned and all vestiges of native culture were in danger of extinction. Children were forced to attend Japanese schools. Use of the Korean language was strictly prohibited. Scholars were jailed and the population was required to worship the Japanese Shinto god. Later, between 100,000 and 200,000 young females were coerced into sexual slavery, acting as "comfort women" for Japanese troops both at home and abroad. Moreover, the Japanese would deceive the poor by using local officials to administer labor quotas essentially pitting Korean against Korean. Thus began one of the darkest periods in Korean history.

The conclusion of hostilities signaling the end of World War I, conjoined with President Woodrow Wilson's doctrine of Fourteen Points espousing self-determination, brought a false glimmer of hope to the oppressed population of Korea. On March 1, 1919, as if instigated by destiny, the nation's elderly Emperor Kojong mysteriously passed away. The general mourning that resulted from this event strangely coincided with the reading of a Declaration of Independence at twelve noon in Seoul's Pagoda Park. This proclamation, penned and read by 33 patriots representing the citizens who had affixed their signatures to the document, ignited a wave of revolutionary fervor throughout the embattled country. Initially personified by demonstrators waving the forbidden national flag and chanting *"taehan tongnip manse"* or "long live Korean independence," the movement spread first throughout Korea and subsequently, the world. The Japanese were quick to act and within three months, 50,000 people were murdered or wounded with others being flogged, jailed, or tortured. In his book titled, *The Truth about Korea*, C.W. Kendall describes the situation by stating: "The horror and brutality of some of the deeds committed are beyond belief." Although unsuccessful for the moment in their bid for independence, this event, which burned a lasting impression in the pages of Korean history, demonstrated the indomitable will of the people and announced to the Japanese in no uncertain terms that force alone could not stem the tide of freedom.

WORLD WAR II AND THE KOREAN CONFLICT

As Europe began to resonate with the rumor of war, Japan continued to exhibit its expansionist policy by invading China, and then aligning itself with Nazi Germany by becoming a signatory of the Axis Pact. Japan's most stunning act of aggression, however, came on Sunday December 7, 1941 when wave after wave of Mitsubishi-built attack aircraft ushered in by the first rays of dawn, descended upon the Pacific Fleet of the United States Navy moored at Pearl Harbor. In responding to this grisly provocation, America finally found herself firmly ensconced in the throes of World War II. As a nation under imperial rule, Korea quickly became a supply depot for Japan's war effort. Koreans of all ages were forced to work in factories and mines, and on military construction projects. In the final days of the conflict when the Japanese began running short of resources, all metal objects including spoons and chopsticks were collected and sent abroad for use in producing munitions. As all hope for a Japanese victory began to wane, cattle and rice production were diverted to Japan as well. On August 15, 1945 Japan finally surrendered to American and Ally forces thus closing the book on 35 years of colonial rule over Korea.

Aside from the devastating effects of the Japanese Occupation and World War II, the single greatest tragedy to befall the Hermit Kingdom in modern times was the Korean Conflict lasting from 1950 to 1953. The stage was unwittingly set for this catastrophic event when a seemingly arbitrary division of land at the 38th parallel allowed Russian and American forces to fill the North and South respectively, essentially relegating the country to an international protectorate. On August 15, 1948, the Republic of Korea was officially inaugurated in the South with Syngman Rhee becoming its first president. A short ten days later, the Democratic People's Republic of Korea was established in the North with Kim Il Sung assuming office as its first leader.

Throughout the 1940s and 1950s, the United Nations played a significant role in determining the ultimate destiny of Korea. In December 1948, the Temporary Commission on Korea recommended that the organization as a whole recognize the R.O.K. as the nation's only legitimate government. Later on, the world body established a committee to oversee the withdrawal of U.S. and Russian occupation forces signaling the final mile on the long road to freedom. However, on June 25, 1950, North Korean Communist forces crossed the 38th parallel and invaded South Korea. The U.N. Security Council recommended that United Nation forces respond. Ultimately, 16 nations heeded the call for assistance with another 40 contributing help in some form. Over the course of the next three years, U.N. and Communist forces battled for superiority over the entire length of the Korean peninsula. Both sides would gain, loose, and reclaim territory. Only on July of 1953 was a tentative truce signed once again establishing the 38th parallel as the official geographical division between North and South Korea. This, the most tenuous of peace agreements creating the world's most heavily armed demilitarized zone, was signed at the cost of hundreds of thousands of Korean lives. For the survivors, there would be no lack of suffering at least in the short term.

Seoul in the mid 1950s was reeling in the aftermath of the Japanese Occupation, World War II, and the Korean War. Homeless orphans in the thousands, whose parents had perished in the trenches, roamed the streets while beggars bereft with affliction searched for opportunities to feed themselves and what remained of their families. Women in truckloads would often use their gender for monetary gain while visiting bases that housed a military that had grown from 100,000 in 1950 to over 600,000 in 1953. Everywhere was squalor and deprivation. In his book, *Korea's Place in the Sun*, historian Bruce Cumings describes the experiences of novelist Ahn Junghyo's parents following the war:

> *My father worked as a carpenter at an American base… and Mother ran a small shop at a nearby intersection at a three-forked road. Everyday I used to go to the garbage dump a little distance off from my house. Often my foot was cut by a used razor blade, on the sharp teeth of a broken saw or a jagged lid of a can, but the cuts were worth it because the whole family could feast on pig soup at dinner if I happened to find a piece of pork among the garbage…Sometimes you would have good fortune and unearth oranges, Hershey chocolate wrapped in sleek brown paper or Brach's jelly candies of five different colors shining like jewels in their cellophane wrappers. One day the American soldiers dumped a heap of chicken legs that had quite a lot of meat still hanging…Mother boiled a delicious soup with those bones and meat and barley, even adding some precious rice. Where had I found all those chicken legs, Father asked me. I told him. That night, he took a rusty tin bucket from the kitchen and asked me to show him the way to the dump.*

Sadly, the horrific conditions affecting Seoul and its people were not unique to the war-torn city. An uprooted agrarian population bearing the baggage of shock and confusion flocked to the cities in search of work leaving no one immune to the ravages of imperial rule and internal strife. All across the nation crime and hunger ran rampant. Is it any wonder then that a nation struggling to revive a golden past wrapped in honor should search its collective consciousness for a remedy representing traditional strengths and values? In short, this was the tragic background against which taekwondo, the traditional martial art of Korea and partial answer to the above quandary, was born.

In concluding this section, I cannot help but recall the emotions I, a foreigner, experienced one sunny, summer morning in 1999 while riding south on the Kyongju Expressway. Gazing out the tinted window of our motor coach, the picturesque scenery could not erase the thought that a few short decades ago the serenity of this now-tranquil place had been shattered by the activities of war. Whether the Communist forces had actually taken this route in pushing the South Koreans back to the apparent safety of the Pusan perimeter was irrelevant at the time. For in doing the research for my last book I knew only too well that the entire country had been indiscriminately soaked with blood in a war between brothers and sisters of the same parent nation. More disturbing, however, was the thought that the onerous division remains to this day with little resolution in sight.

CHAPTER 3

The Formative Years of Taekwondo

THE CRUCIBLE OF CREATION / THE KWANS

The turbulent years that spanned the first half of the twentieth century found many Korean martial artists whose lives were in jeopardy by virtue of their art, emigrating to Japan or China where they were assigned work or worse, conscripted to serve the very military machine that was actively crushing their homeland. Here in these foreign lands, Korean masters were not only permitted to practice the martial arts forbidden by imperial rule back home, but to earn advancement and teaching credentials as well. Pivotal figures such as General Choi, Hong Hi, Won Kuk Lee and Hwang Kee were beneficiaries of this dubious yet practical historical aberration. Borrowing from a variety of provincial styles, these pioneers and others would later return to Korea then under a different sort of domination albeit more benign, to launch or create martial arts and enduring organizations of their own with a distinctly Korean flavor yet colored by cultural impressions and methods accumulated abroad.

Compiling an accurate history of this period, when taekwondo, was in its formative stages, is difficult at best given the erratic nature of its documentation. Major occurrences were seldom committed to paper and when they were, risked destruction at the hands of opposing forces. To this day, aside from articles appearing on the worldwide web, in academic journals and in magazines, history and tradition continues to be transmitted by word of mouth and martial actions that date back to antiquity. At the center of this chronological confusion is the creation of the various martial art schools that evolved during the chaotic 1940s and 1950s. These schools came to be known as the *kwans* and the story of their similarities, differences, founders and politics, is pivotal to the birth of traditional taekwondo. It is a story that few know in totality and even fewer have researched sufficiently to document accurately. Unfortunately, the scope of this book will not permit an in-depth exploration of this topic since its focus is heavily weighted towards defensive strategy rather then a comprehensive history. However, because of the significance of this tale, an attempt will be made in the future to seek out those familiar with this period and, through their personal experiences, piece together a cohesive picture of those times in written form. For now, a perfunctory investigation will have to suffice.

Most sources concur that at least five and possibly six *kwans* were created prior to and shortly following the collapse of Japanese rule. These included the Chung Do Kwan, Moo Duk Kwan, Yun Moo Kwan, Song Moo Kwan, Chang Moo Kwan and Kuk Moo Kwan. Others followed shortly after.

Table of the Original Kwans

Kwan Name	Established	Founder
Chung Do Kwan	1944	Won Kuk Lee
Song Moo Kwan	1944	Byong Jik No
Moo Duk Kwan	1945	Hwang Kee
Yun Moo Kwan	1946	Sang Sup Chun
Chang Moo Kwan	1947	Byung In Yoon
Kuk Moo Kwan	1949	Suh Chong Kang

Since the term "taekwondo" had yet to be coined, the disciplines practiced during this period went under the monikers of *tae soo do* (kick, fist, Way), *tang soo do* (Way of the China hand), *kong soo do* (Way of the empty hand) and *kwonbop* (Way of the fist).

One of the first to establish a stable Korean training venue was Won Kuk Lee, born on April 13, 1907.

While at university, Lee began his formal training in Japan under Gichin Funakoshi, a student of Yasutsune Itosu whom we shall meet later in this book. There he claims to have studied the Korean martial arts forbidden by law back home. Lee bolstered his martial arts education by visiting various training centers in Okinawa and China during his travels abroad. This exposure resulted in his becoming a student of Shotokan karate-do.

After returning to Korea in 1944, Lee twice sought permission from the occupation government to teach his countrymen native martial arts. This was possible only because the Japanese had lifted the ban on defensive training in 1943. Following an initial refusal, Lee ultimately was given the nod to proceed and began teaching at the Yung Shin School in the Ok Chun Dong district. As we have seen, Seoul at this time was a hotbed of unrest. Gangs and political groups roamed the streets at will often resorting to the use of martial arts in the resolution of conflict. In response, the imperial forces, enjoying their final days in power, again clamped down on martial arts instruction in public buildings. A man not to be deterred, Won Kuk Lee went on to establish what was to become the preeminent martial arts academy of the time choosing the name Chung Do Kwan, or the "Blue Wave Institute".

Lee secured quarters for his training hall at Ya Go Sa Temple, but was later forced to relocate several times, eventually settling at Number 80 in the Kyun Ji Dong district of Seoul. Sung Duk Son eventually assumed the leading role following Lee's retirement later followed by Woon Kyu Uhm.

Likewise, Hwang Kee, the originator of *soo bahk do moo duk kwan*, born on November 9, 1914, was the recipient of a similar amalgamation of styles.

In 1921 at age seven, Kee became enthralled with the martial arts when he witnessed an attack on a lone man by a group of ruffians. Relying on a series of blocks and kicks, the outnumbered defender eventually defeated his aggressors. This display of fighting skill so impressed the future grandmaster that he immediately dedicated himself to a

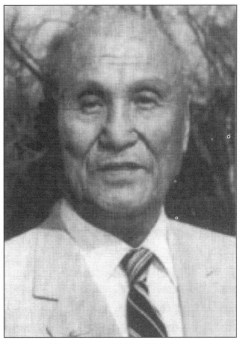

Grandmaster Won Kuk Lee, founder of the Chung Do Kwan.

diligent study of the martial arts. Despite the existing Japanese prohibition on martial arts training, Kee practiced in secret mastering the native defensive styles of *taekkyon* and *subak*, the art of punching, kicking, and butting, yet another Korean combat discipline with roots deep in antiquity. In 1936, the discovery of his clandestine training by the occupying forces earned him jail time and a death sentence. Having escaped his detractors, Kee packed what belongings he had and went on to study Chinese martial arts while employed as a railroad worker in Manchuria. Under the watchful eye of Master Yang Kuk Jin, Kee gained instruction in *she bop* (postures), *bo bop* (steps), *ryun bop* (conditioning), and *hyung* (forms).

On November 9, 1945, after returning to Seoul, he established the Moo Duk Kwan or the "Institute of Martial Virtue."

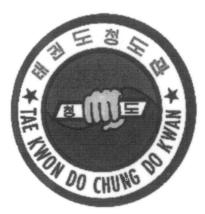

Chung Do Kwan emblem.

It was here that Kee began teaching *soo bahk do*, a martial art that to this day exhibits strong Chinese overtones. *Soo bahk do* is a relatively new martial art developed by Grandmaster Hwang Kee following his discovery of the *Muye Dobo-Tongji*; a written collection of native martial arts techniques dating back to the Yi (Chosun) Dynasty.

Taekkyon, the circular kicking art, was still popular at the time regardless of the fact that gang members were busily corrupting its defensive nature by using it as a form of physical harassment against their fellow citizens. Despite this unfortunate use of the discipline, on September 1, 1946, Grandmaster Byung In Yoon founded a taekkyon club at the Kyung Sung Agricultural High School in Seoul. Raised in Manchuria, Yoon studied chuan fa before attending college at Nihon University in Tokyo during the 1940s. There he made the acquaintance of Grandmaster

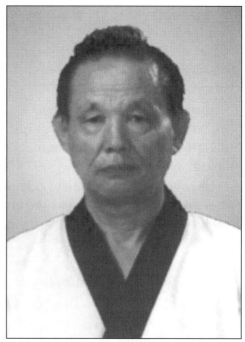

Grandmaster Hwang Kee, founder of the Moo Duk Kwan.

Kanken Toyama, founder of Shudokan karate and a member of the University's collegium. The two accomplished practitioners shared their knowledge of the martial arts with Toyama eventually promoting Yoon to the rank of fourth degree black belt. Yoon later established the Chang Moo Kwan or "Martial Spirit Training Institute" at the Seoul YMCA naming Nam Suk Lee as his first instructor.

The difficult times Koreans were experiencing affected everyone and the *kwans* were not immune. Many students were called up for military service causing great losses in enrollment. Sadly, by the time the Korean War had ended, Byung In Yoon was missing and considered killed. Nam Suk Lee assumed the role of *kwanjangnim*, or head of the institute. Under his leadership, the Chang Moo Kwan flourished becoming the preeminent *dojang* in Seoul for self-

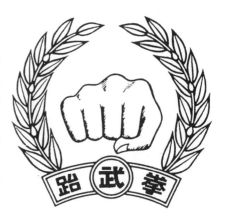

Moo Duk Kwan Tae Kwon Do emblem.

defense. Later, in 1965, in what can be construed as an effort to expand on his success, Lee extricated his organization from the Korea Taekwondo Association and formed the World Chang Moo Kwan Taekwondo Association. While Nam Suk Lee died on August 29, 2000, his vision proved worthwhile with many affiliate schools currently practicing Chang Moo Kwan Taekwondo worldwide.

It was not unusual during this period for additional *kwans* to develop as a subset of other, better established schools. This was certainly the case with the Oh Do Kwan which we shall examine shortly, and to a lesser degree, the Kuk Moo Kwan.

Created in 1949 by Suh Chong Kang, the Kuk Moo Kwan, or "National Martial Arts Institute," was located in Incheon. During the Japanese Occupation, Kang was one of a select group of students who secretly trained with Won Kuk Lee at the Chung Do Kwan. The reputation of this style seems to have revolved around the abilities of its creator; in charge of a student militia during the Korean War, he managed on several occasions to escape from his captors by relying on his martial arts skills. Later, in 1955, Suh Chong Kang was appointed director of the HID, the Korean military intelligence agency, by General Choi, Hong Hi. His duties included overseeing defensive positions around Incheon and the training of spies meant to infiltrate the North. After eleven years in the service of his country, Kang went on to become the head instructor for the Incheon police department while teaching his style of martial arts at various military installations to Korean armed forces bound for Vietnam. Declining an Ambassadorship to Malaysia in 1968, he instead immigrated to America to insure the formal education of his sons who carry on the Kuk Moo Kwan tradition today.

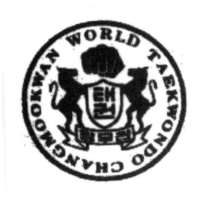

Chang Moo Kwan emblem.

Some schools, at least initially given their location and the living conditions in Korea at the time, were not as successful as others in their ability to maintain a working student base. One such school was the Sang Moo Kwan or the "Ever Youthful Institute of Martial Arts".

Established on March 11, 1944 in Kaesong, its founder Byung Jik Ro was born on July 3, 1919. Intrigued as a youth when he witnessed martial arts being practiced at local temples, he subsequently sought out the instruction of Gichin Funakoshi in 1936 while attending college in Japan. In 1944, after earning his black belt, Ro returned to Kaesong and developed supplementary techniques that provided a foundation for the curriculum that would be unique to the Sang Moo Kwan. His first attempt to open a *dojang* at the Kwan Duk Jung archery school proved futile and he was forced to close after only four months. In May of 1946, another effort was made but resulted in closure as well forcing the students of the Song Moo Kwan to abandon their dreams yet again. With an enormous show of the indomitable will so prevalent in the Korean people, Ro again opened the Sang Moo Kwan in 1953. This time he and his instructors were triumphant partially due to the abundance of foreign troops that remained in the country following the war. Not only did these soldiers practice the martial arts locally, but continued their training after returning home to their native lands thus spreading the art taught at the Sang Moo Kwan even further. In the same year, Byung Jik Ro became executive director of the newly established Korea Kong Soo Do Association, a predecessor to the KTA, and was elemental in unifying the kwans that eventually supported the defensive art of that came to be known as taekwondo in the 1950's.

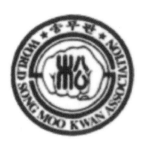

Song Moo Kwan emblem.

A predecessor to the Ji Do Kwan, or the "Wisdom Way Institute", the Yun Moo Kwan was established on May 3, 1946 in the Soo Song Dong district of Seoul. Its founder, Sang Sup Chun, studied both judo and karate while in school. At the commencement of the Korea War in 1950, Chun was abducted and believed to have been taken to North Korea where he was killed. Following Chun's disappearance, the Yun Moo Kwan closed, but later emerged as the Ji Do Kwan under the direction of Kwe Byung Yoon and Chong Woo Lee, two of Chun's students. The Ji Do Kwan, as would other well established martial arts schools of this era, go on to unite under government supervision and spin off students that would change the complexion of the Korean martial arts forever.

GENERAL CHOI, HONG HI

Perhaps the most visible protagonist in the evolutionary process of taekwondo was General Choi, Hong Hi who in the 1930s began his training under Hong Il Dong. Hong not only taught his young student calligraphy but also, due to his frail nature, began teaching him *taekkyon*, the indigenous martial discipline unique to the Korean peninsula. In 1937, the future "father of taekwondo" was sent to Kyoto to further his education. There he met a Korean instructor and, following a regimen of intense training, earned a first-degree black belt in karate. Later, after settling in Tokyo, he continued his training under the direction of Master Gichin Funakoshi, founder of Shotokan karate-do, while attending the Law School of Choong Ang University. After being promoted to second-degree black belt, Choi and his friend Byung In Yoon began teaching karate at the Tokyo YMCA.

During this period in his life, Choi was forced to join the Japanese military. Realizing how little hope there was of a victory over the United States and its allies, he and thirty other students attempted to escape to the Baekdoo Mountains on the Manchurian-Korea border. There they hoped to link up with the Korean Liberation Army and offer resistance to the forces occupying their homeland. His attempt failed, however, and he was arrested and tried for treason. Choi, whose

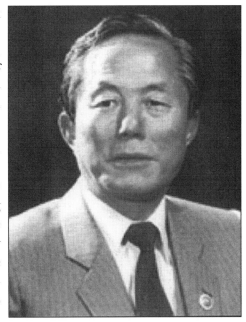

General Choi, Hong Hi, founder of the Oh-Do Kwan and the International Taekwondo Federation.

original sentence called for a seven-year prison term, was later condemned to be executed on August 18, 1945. Three days prior to his execution, Japan surrendered to Allied forces and on August 15, 1945, Choi found himself a free man.

Following his release, Choi quickly ascended through the ranks of the Korean military where he became an instructor for the American Military Police stationed in Seoul. In 1949, General Choi was responsible for staging the first *kong soo do* demonstration in the United States while training at Fort Riley, Kansas. Shortly after in 1952, the Korean martial arts received a significant boost in popularity following a demonstration staged for President Syngman Rhee. So impressed was he by the proficiency and effectiveness of the practitioners involved that he ordered all soldiers to begin training in the martial arts. Consequently, in 1953 General Choi, Hong Hi created the 29th Infantry Division at the request of the chief of

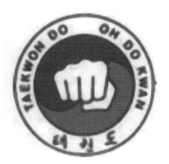

Oh Do Kwan emblem.

staff of the Korean Army, General Sun Yub Baek. Symbolized by the insignia depicting a fist over the Korean peninsula, the "Fist" or Il Keu Division distinguished itself by marrying regulation drills with martial arts training making it a truly unique entity within the Korean military.

According to General Choi, his soldiers were "ready to fight with or without weapons." At the same time, the General founded a training academy within the military that came to be known as the Oh Do Kwan or "Institute of My Way."

Empty hand, Korean defensive strategy had now been crystallized within the armed forces. Furthermore, General Choi is rightly credited with developing much of what we know today as traditional taekwondo along with its unique set of *tul*, or forms, known as the *Chang-Han* series; originally a set of twenty *hyung* with four additional forms being added in the 1970s. This development was a direct result of his contempt for the Japanese and the desire to spawn a martial art with a distinctly Korean philosophy. However, his contribution to taekwondo, coupled with that of other courageous innovators, as we shall see, did not stop there.

As far back as 1946, attempts were made to unify the Korean martial arts while eliminating foreign influences that were injected during the Japanese Occupation. However, if any date can be recognized as the birthday of taekwondo it would, in all likelihood, be April 11, 1955. It was on this day that an influential group of men sat in conference with the purpose of uniting and proposing a name for the loose confederation of Korean disciplines that would come to be known as *taekwondo*.

Among them were Yoo Hwa Chung, Son Duk Sung, Gen. Choi, Hong Hi, Gen. Lee Hyung Ku, Cho Kyung Kyu, Chung Dae Chun, Han Chang Won, Chang Kyung Rok, Hong Soon Ho, Ko Kwang Rae, and Hyun Jong Myung. Some were martial artists; others, financiers, politicians, and military men. A record of this meeting states, "Choi recommends the name *taekwondo*. He explains the name both literally and technically. Mr. Yoo says, "I completely agree with the name *taekwon* submitted by General Choi. I think, however, it would be utterly significant that we have the approval from the president, Syngman Rhee, since giving a name to a martial art is so important." All members unanimously agreed."

In spite of this evidence, the naming of the internationally recognized Korean martial art to this day remains surrounded by controversy. Other notable figures, including Won Kuk Lee, also lay claim to its inception. However, most historians agree that it was General Choi who first labeled the art. Choi purportedly coined the name taekwondo based the fact that his comprehensive system emphasized the use of both kicking and punching, and bore a striking resemblance to the traditional art of *taekkyon*. Oddly enough, upon consideration President Rhee at first rejected the

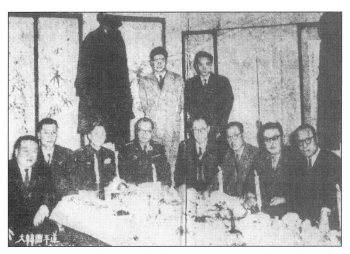

April 11, 1955 photograph of naming ceremony for Taekwondo.

name, preferring instead the actual term *taekkyon* with its nostalgic connection to the past. Choi appealed to his colleagues, the president's Chief of Staff Kwak Young Joo, and Suh Jung Huk, director of the Presidential Protection Forces. He explained that his was an original syllabus, different from that of its traditional companion. Choi requested that they use their proximity to the Korean leader in persuading him to accept the new name. Rhee, as fate would have it, acquiesced. Choi was quick to act, directing that signs bearing the name *tang soo do* be removed from Oh Do Kwan and Chung Do Kwan locations and replaced by those proudly announcing the name of the newly unified Korean martial art. These events, however, did not negate the fact that for many years following, masters of competing *dojangs* or schools, refused to recognize the recently adopted imprimatur.

In the autumn of 1959, Choi once again called a meeting of the existing *kwan* leaders, this time to recommend unification and admittance into the Korea Sports Union (KSU), an alliance that already included judo and kumdo practitioners. Nevertheless, by his own admission, the General had originally intended to create an entity of his own that would stand in contrast to the competition-based organizations of the day. This coalition was to be called the Korea Martial Arts Association whose primary mission would be to emphasize the philosophical component of taekwondo. In all likelihood, Choi realized that membership in this sports-oriented body would support the position of taekwondo in the eyes of those reluctant to see things his way, and so his vision, in its pure form, never materialized. In attendance at this gathering was Byung Jik No representing the Song Moo Kwan, Kwe Byung Yoon of the Ji

Do Kwan, Nam Suk Lee of the Chang Moo Kwan, and Hwang Kee on behalf of the Moo Duk Kwan. Choi, himself, spoke for the Oh Do Kwan and Chung Do Kwan. He explained that in order to gain membership in the KSU, one common title for their martial art was required. Friction erupted during the discussion with Lee, No and Kee insisting on the continued use of the term *tang soo do*. Following a heated debate, Choi claims he convinced his guests to once again accept the name *taekwondo*. A hierarchal structure for this new organization was agreed upon and officers were elected with General Choi, Hong Hi becoming the first president of the newly created, Korea Taekwondo Association.

This success, however, was short lived. On April 19, 1960, a student uprising resulted in the overthrow of the Rhee government. Recognition of the Korea Taekwondo Association was put on hold.

Following a military coup d'etat in 1961 that resulted in the installation of Chung Hee Park as President of South Korea, General Choi, Hong Hi was appointed Ambassador to Malaysia. Prior to his departure, he again attempted registration with the Korea Sports Union. Another meeting was convened to consider terms of membership since by now a new generation of masters had assumed leadership roles within the *kwans*. The discussion centered on a name for their mutual organization. Reminding the assemblage that the term taekwondo had already been chosen, Choi left the gathering in a state of frustration. Removed somewhat from the political arena due to his responsibilities abroad and thus unable to express his influence directly, the name of the alliance Choi founded evolved yet again to the Korea Tae Soo Do Association.

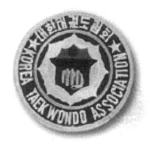

Upon his return to Korea in 1965, General Choi observed that the rules governing *tae soo do* competitions sadly mirrored those of Japanese karate. At a conference of the General Assembly, Choi announced that a change was necessary both in regulation and in name and called for the term taekwondo to be reinstated. Following a vote, his wish was realized by a single ballot. Once again, General Choi, Hong Hi found himself president

Korea Taekwondo Association emblem.

of the revived Korea Taekwondo Association. During his tenure, Choi traveled throughout Asia and Europe spreading knowledge of taekwondo. Acting as team leader to Kyo Cha Han, Jong Soo Park, Jae Hwa Kwan, and Joong Keun Kim, he arranged and presented frequent demonstrations depicting the effectiveness of his native discipline.

Finally, on March 22, 1966, representatives from a variety of nations met with Choi resulting in taekwondo assuming its rightful place as a global martial art with the founding of the International Taekwon-Do Federation (ITF). What began as a group of nine charter members including Korea, Malaysia, Vietnam, Singapore, West Germany, America, Egypt, Italy, and Turkey, quickly grew to a worldwide organization boasting thirty members in two years. Yet unfortunately, even taekwondo, complete with its honorable and virtuous background is not immune to internal politics. Choi eventually fell out of grace with the Korean government in part due to his insistence on demonstrating taekwondo in North Korea, and immigrated to Canada taking the workings of the International Taekwon-Do Federation (ITF) along with him. While this organization flourished and continues to maintain a strong global presence, the torch of constant progress, at least in Korea, the homeland of taekwondo, was handed on to yet another leader of equal foresight and vigor.

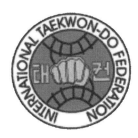

International Taekwon-Do Federation emblem.

DR. UN YONG KIM, "DRAGON ABOVE THE CLOUDS"

If it can be said that General Choi, Hong Hi was accountable for the early growth of traditional taekwondo, then it would be equally correct to say that Dr. Un Yong Kim, is responsible for the explosive acceptance of taekwondo as a world sport. Born on March 19, 1931 in Seoul, Korea, Kim served his country on the battlefield during the Korean War. In 1956, Un Yong, literally translated as "dragon above the clouds", graduated from Texas Western College in the United States, after satisfying a yearning to master the Spanish and English languages. Yet, as was the case with many young Korean men of his time, he dreamed of becoming a diplomat in the service of his native land and so he returned to Korea. In 1965, two years after receiving his doctorate from Yonsei University, this ambition was fully realized when he was appointed representative to the 20th United Nations General Assembly.

In 1967, while serving at the United Nations, Dr. Kim made a major contribution the American martial arts community. He, along with General James Van Fleet, an adjunct of General Douglas MacArthur, approached Master Richard Chun, one of the five original instructors along with Ki Whang Kim, Daeshik Kim, Sijak Henry Cho and Jhoon Rhee, to immigrate to America in the 1960s, about organizing a

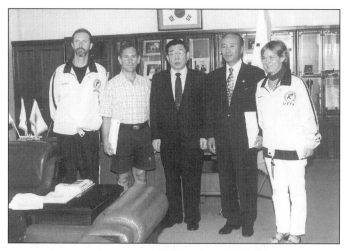

Dr. Un Yong Kim (center) with Grandmaster Richard Chun and
Master Doug Cook (far left) at the Kukkiwon in Seoul, South Korea.

competitive event unlike any other seen before. It would be known as the First Universal Open Championship. Aside from promoting Korean culture to the American public at large, the proposed tournament would feature a spectrum of fighters from Japanese and Chinese disciplines as well as the obvious Korean stylists; something that had not been done previously. The event proved to be a great success with over two thousand spectators and four hundred fifty participants vying to place. What began as an isolated competition evolved into an annual event that lasted a full decade through the concerted efforts of Dr. Kim and Grandmaster Chun.

Over the years, Dr. Kim would frequently employ Richard Chun to act on his behalf as an instrument of the World Taekwondo Federation (WTF) in America. Since Grandmaster Chun has played such a significant role in promoting traditional taekwondo in the United States and the world through his ties to the WTF and Dr. Kim, it is worth retrogressing for a moment to examine a few of his accomplishments.

Born in 1935 in Seoul, Richard Chun studied under Master Chong Soo Hong at the famed Moo Duk Kwan Institute. He advanced quickly through the ranks after demonstrating great proficiency in the art, but was forced to interrupt his training when his family fled to Cheju Island during the Korean War. Determined to remain faithful to his practice, Grandmaster Chun continued through the execution of a series of solo, choreographed self-defense movements known as *poom-se*, high in the mountains overlooking his new home. To this day Grandmaster Chun remains an avid believer in the importance of forms.

After receiving a degree at Yonsei University, Un Yong Kim's alma mater, Chun decided to leave his native land to teach practitioners living in the United States traditional martial arts skills. There he went on to earn a doctorate in physical education, launch the Richard Chun Taekwondo Center in New York City, and establish the United States Taekwondo Association (USTA) whose mission it is to "promote the ancient and evolving art of taekwondo." In 1999, ten years after receiving his ninth dan from the World Taekwondo Federation, Grandmaster Chun was appointed Special Assistant to Dr. Un Yong Kim.

While remaining in government service, Dr. Kim, an accomplished concert pianist and polyglot, fluent in five languages, increasingly began focusing on sports. In 1971, he became president of the Korea Taekwondo Association and, in 1972, was awarded the "Korea Sports Prize".

In 1973, the future of taekwondo was to become indelibly stamped with the vision and actions of Dr. Un Yong Kim when he was named president of the World Taekwondo Federation; a position he would hold for over thirty years.

In a statement for an interview written by Kang Seok Lee for *Tae Kwon Do Times* magazine, Dr. Kim's enthusiasm for the sport of taekwondo was evident when he said: "The Olympic Festival promotes a combination of culture, sports and education; a friendlier world, peace, unity, and a

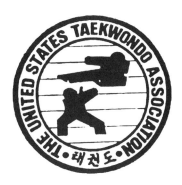

United States Taekwondo Association emblem.

better quality of life. The finest athletes from around the world gather to exchange ideas and compete at an elite level. Many of these youths will be responsible for our future."

Dr. Kim's magnanimous character manifested itself whenever taekwondo practitioners from foreign lands would visit the World Taekwondo Federation headquarters housed at the *Kukkiwon* in Seoul. Taking time out from an extraordinarily busy schedule that would often cause an absence from his family for nine months out of the year, he would meet with them as he did with our group in 1999, to deliver an inspiring dissertation regarding the past, present and future of taekwondo.

THE WORLD TAEKWONDO FEDERATION AND THE KUKKIWON

Following his election as president of the Korea Taekwondo Association in 1971, Dr. Kim and others felt the need for a centralized training facility where practitioners from around the globe could gather collectively to train, test, and seek advance-

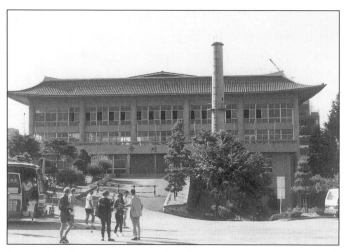

The Kukkiwon. Seoul, South Korea. Built to follow traditional Korean architecture.

ment in the art of taekwondo. His efforts resulted in the building of the Kukkiwon, now the Mecca of taekwondo operations worldwide.

Literally translated as "National Gymnasium", the Kukkiwon is located atop a hillside in the Kangnam District of Seoul. Construction began on November 9, 1971 with the facility being inaugurated on November 30, 1972. Mirroring traditional Korean architecture, its humble exterior is deceptive in that it houses management offices, locker rooms, seminar space, and a museum. However, perhaps most importantly, aside from the large competition area that allows various national and university teams to test their skills against one another, until recently it was headquarters to the Secretariat of the World Taekwondo Federation (WTF) established on June 3, 1973. This organization effectively replaced the International Taekwon-Do Federation (ITF), the brainchild, as we have seen of General Choi, Hong Hi. Its origination was precipitated following a meeting of the thirty delegate countries that had participated in the First World Taekwondo Championships held at the Kukkiwon in May of 1973. At this meeting Dr. Un Yong Kim was elected president of the new federation.

Presently, the World Taekwondo Federation in unison with the Kukkiwon, acts as a clearinghouse for the many applicants throughout the world seeking legitimate black belt certification through their national governing bodies or NGB's. Oddly enough, one would assume that such noble institutions would, at least in part, be subsidized by the Korean government. The majority of funding, however, is received through the issuance of the aforementioned dan, or black belt grade, certifications.

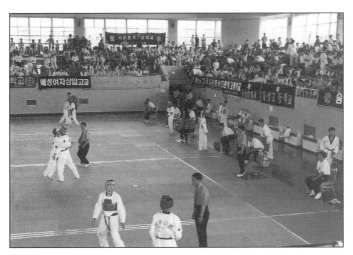

Korean taekwondo practitioners compete at the Kukkiwon.

The WTF, as with any complex organization, is composed of many committees. The Technical Committee is responsible for maintaining traditional technique as well as developing modern, innovative methods of competition. Additional entities such as the Financial, Women's, Collegiate and Referee Committees oversee specialized concentrations within the organization. Moreover, practitioners from every corner of the globe visit the Taekwondo Academy housed at the Kukkiwon to take advantage of the comprehensive Instructor Program available to advanced students. Standing on the highly polished, wooden floor of this dynamic monument to taekwondo is an awe inspiring experience to say the least. One cannot help but sense the spirit and energy of the many dedicated Korean martial artists who have devoted their lives to making taekwondo an Olympic sport and a highly standardized system of self-defense.

A WORLD SPORT / THE OLYMPICS

In 1988, a monumental event took place that solidified taekwondo as a world sport in the eyes of the general public. To the delight of its citizenry, Seoul, South Korea played host to the 1988 Olympic Games.

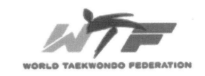

Since the country chosen to sponsor the event is traditionally entitled to choose a demonstration sport, the Korean leadership, including Dr. Kim, who had become Vice President of the Seoul Olympic Organizing Committee and a member

World Taekwondo Federation emblem.

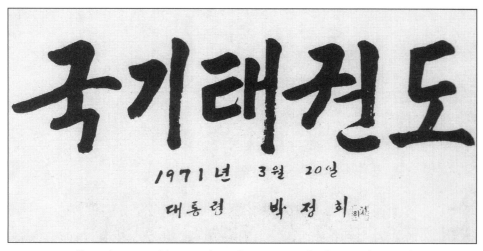

Calligraphy created by President Chung Hee Park of Korea that reads:
"A National Sport, Taekwondo."

of the International Olympic Committee by 1986, naturally chose to display taekwondo with great success. Row upon row of seasoned taekwondo practitioners performed basic techniques and breaking skills on the field of the newly built Olympic Stadium that was filled to capacity. This honor united the hearts and minds of the Korean people and catapulted their national martial art to world prominence.

Dr. Un Yong Kim, who in 1992 became vice president of the International Olympic Committee, continued promoting taekwondo on an international level through his affiliation with various sports organizations. Named an Executive Board Member of the IOC in 1997, it is largely due to Dr. Kim's untiring efforts that taekwondo debuted at the 2000 Sydney Olympics as a full-medal Olympic sport and then again in the 2004 Athens games.

Yet, as virtuous as taekwondo is intended to be, sadly, it is not immune from the politics so often prevalent today in government, business, and society at large. In 2004, after more than three decades of service, Dr. Un Yong Kim was forced to abandon his post as the de facto leader of sport taekwondo and step down amidst a cloud of allegations accusing him of wrongdoing.

Succeeded by Dr. Cungwon Choue as president of the World Taekwondo Federation, and Woon Kyu Uhm, an original member of the Chung Do Kwan as president of the Kukkiwon, the future participation of taekwondo as an Olympic event was suddenly thrown into doubt. However, as of this writing, sport taekwondo, along with judo, will once again share the honor of being the only two Asian martial arts with competitors vying to place at the 2008 Olympic Games in Beijing, China.

TAEKWONDO IN THE NEW MILLENNIUM

While the historical perspective submitted above is not intended to be a definitive narrative on the history of taekwondo and Korea, its nation of origin, it does attempt to explain a modicum of the controversies, intrigues, heartbreaks, and accomplishments that, over the course of time, have rendered a loosely knit group of native fighting styles into a single, cohesive martial art and international sport with, at the turn of the millennium, over sixty-million students practicing worldwide.

Still, given the information gathered so far, one may ask, what does the future have in store for taekwondo and how does it fit in the mosaic of spiritual pursuits so prevalent today? Will it evolve into nothing more than a combat sport, or will it retain the philosophical underpinnings and defensive value that validate it as a traditional martial art? Before moving on, let us for a moment consider these issues.

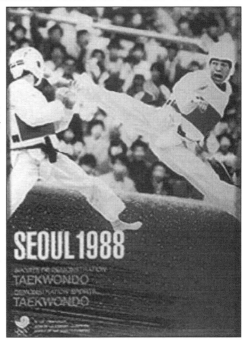

The dawning of the twenty-first century has seen much in the way of conflict both on a global and personal level. More than ever, cultural differences coupled with opposing worldviews appear to have spiraled out of control. The integrity of our most sacred institutions has been brought into question with internal corruption tearing at the roots of government, big business, and even religion. More than ever, we find ourselves turning inside for answers. For decades, traditional taekwondo has been the perfect medium for cultivating inner strength, extraordinary endurance, and an effective arsenal of defensive skills. In its current iteration it can be thought of as a direct reflection of modern society's desire for a ritualized discipline devoid of religious dogma, but complete with a physically and spiritually enhanced set of ethical principles by which to live. Consequently, motives for training in the martial arts today range anywhere from gaining proficiency in self-defense and physical fitness, to propagating discipline and focus in adolescent children that might otherwise be glued to a television set or computer screen. There is little doubt that practitioners of all ages can profit greatly from

1988 Olympics Taekwondo poster.

a sincere study of traditional taekwondo.

While sports and all its trappings can provide an outlet for aggression and create social bonds by way of teambuilding, it is, by definition restricted to a set place and time. Likewise, while organized religion attempts to satisfy an innate desire for spiritual enlightenment, it does nothing to address the physical needs of the individual. Martial arts, on the other hand, at least in this author's opinion, if offered in a traditional manner, represent a way of life and a vehicle for self-enrichment through diligent training. Invariably, one will ask how a pursuit so resonant with aggressive overtones can benefit humanity. The solution to this paradox can be found in the realization that the more frequently one trains and becomes proficient in the martial arts, the more one discovers that they have less to defend against. Confidence begins to replace fear. Defensive skills become internalized resulting in one's ability to walk life's path appreciating its simple pleasures rather than being blinded by its daily perils. Now more than ever, these benefits reflect the true worth of taekwondo training.

With roots dating back to antiquity, the robust philosophical foundation that acted as a code of honor for the Hwarang of ancient Silla continues to support traditional taekwondo in the new millennium and remains as valid today as it was in the seventh century when these noble warriors sought ethical wisdom beyond the field of battle.

Student Creed of Taekwondo

- Be loyal to your country
- Be loving and show fidelity to your parents
- Be loving between husband and wife
- Be cooperative between brothers and sisters
- Be faithful to your friends
- Be respectful to your elders
- Establish trust between teacher and student
- Use good judgment before harming any living thing
- Never retreat in battle
- Always finish what you start

Five Tenets of Taekwondo

English	Korean
Courtesy	Ye Ui
Integrity	Yom Chi
Perseverance	In Nae
Self-Control	Guk Gi
Indomitable Spirit	Baekjul Boolgool

Certainly, Buddhism, and to a lesser degree, Taoism, served as the cornerstones of this philosophy. Nevertheless, as we have seen, it was Confucianism, with its blueprint rooted in ethical behavior that flourished during the Chosun Dynasty (1392-1910), manifesting itself in a grand form on the social fabric of Korea. Bearing this in mind, even now we can witness the value of this ethical paradigm when applied to our daily routine.

Confucius taught that a single individual can influence world events through the simple projection of a benevolent state of mind. The Korean proverb, *Su shin je ga chi guk pyong chun fa*, supports this notion, once again confirming the vital role Confucianism played in molding the cultural landscape of the Korean nation. Loosely translated, this dictum states, "Peace within the individual brings peace within the family; peace in the family brings peace in the community; peace in the community, peace in the country and peace throughout the world." As improbable as this may sound, there is little doubt that compassion towards fellow human beings goes a long way. Rather than being isolated in a vacuum, correct action ripples across humanity with the same effect, as would a pebble when dropped into a serene pool of water. While we are certain to encounter speed bumps of belligerency on our path to fulfillment, we must recall that, by and large, a great majority of our fellow human beings desire peace, prosperity and understanding as much as we do. Given this what better way to initiate the reaffirmation of these principles than within ourselves using the ethical doctrine of traditional taekwondo as a roadmap.

Unquestionably, taekwondo is about kicking, striking, and self-defense. Moreover, it has blossomed into a world sport with full recognition by the International Olympic Committee. Yet, in the twenty-first century, as in the past, it remains a vehicle for developing a strong character and a sharp mind. One is constantly reminded of this dichotomy by the universal symbol of the Um/Yang (Yin/Yang in Chinese, In/Yo in Japanese) that vividly depicts the natural harmony between contrasting opposites.

stantly reminded of this dichotomy by the universal symbol of the Um/Yang (Yin/Yang in Chinese, In/Yo in Japanese) that vividly depicts the natural harmony between contrasting opposites.

The sincere taekwondoist actively attempts to cultivate these virtues through a regimen of diligent practice and a pursuit of the Way; however, this is no easy chore given the distractions that often envelop us like a whirlwind. In order to be successful at this task, we must remain mindful of the pitfalls we encounter on a daily basis and apply the ethical training we receive through taekwondo wherever and to whomever it applies.

Ultimately, the martial artist of the new millennium should not only be physically fit and adroit in the ways of self-defense, but in addition, become a beacon of strength and courage for family, friends and those less fortunate than he or she. The above, amplified by an element of self-respect and proficiency in self-defense, is what it means to be a true modern day warrior clad in the armor of virtuous action tailored by a earnest study of traditional taekwondo.

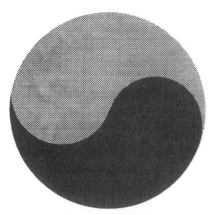

The Korean Um/Yang.

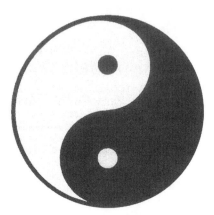

The Chinese Yin/Yang.

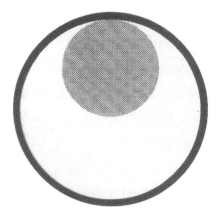

The Japanese In/Yo.

PART TWO

Philosophy

CHAPTER 4

The Role of Meditation in Traditional Taekwondo

The preparatory exercises discussed in this chapter identify traditional taekwondo as a holistic martial art and differentiate it significantly from taekwondo, the world sport. In disciplines other than the martial arts such as yoga, meditation is used as a means of relaxation. In Zen Buddhism, it is used as a vehicle towards enlightenment or *zazen*. However, in traditional taekwondo, meditation is practiced in the hope of calming the restless winds that buffet the mind, to stoke the fires of the universal life force, and to prepare the spirit for the rigors of self-defense. Physically, it relaxes musculature thus decreasing the body's physical response time. Emotionally, it removes the many hurdles that encumber concentration. Still, this essential training element is often overlooked except in schools addressing the more traditional aspects of taekwondo.

Observing a martial artist seated quietly in a *seiza* or meditative posture bears little resemblance to the skilled defender most assume him to be. Meditation, however, plays a vital role in preparing the taekwondoist, both mentally and spiritually, for the demands of self-defense coupled with the essential development and channeling of *Ki*, the universal life force. Moreover, the act of meditation represents a spiritual boundary between the distractions of daily life and the focused mind one requires in the training hall. At the command of *myuk sang*, the taekwondoist trains his body to filter out extraneous thoughts that will interfere with technique.

To begin with, in order to respond rapidly in the face of a threat that has escalated beyond verbal mediation, the mind and the body must react rather than anticipate. This important distinction lies at the core of traditional defensive strategy. Making the false assumption that an attacker will execute a reverse punch when, in truth, his intention is to kick, may result in severe injury to the defender. To appreciate the value of meditation as it applies to this component of self-defense, one needs look no further than the stillness of a serene pool of water reflecting the image of a full moon. Because the surface is unbroken by ripples, the image is pure and undistorted. The mind of the martial artist can be taught to act in a similar fashion.

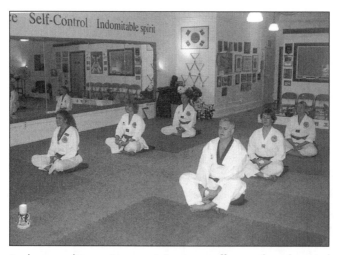

Students meditate prior to training in an effort to clear the mind.

Through the sincere and diligent practice of meditation, the taekwondoist will develop an uncanny ability to react to an unprovoked attack rather than anticipate a potentially false move. How is this possible?

The mind, like an unbroken stallion, has a proclivity for galloping away when left to its own designs. Thoughts of daily activities, bills, work, or school, all have the ability to intrude on a tranquil mind. Great effort is required to focus on…nothing. Yes, it is true. Nothing, no mind, or *mushin*, is what the martial artist seeks. *Mushin* is the mental state where one is unhindered by preconception. As difficult as this stage of consciousness may be to achieve, we do have an ally in our quest. Just as the Asian warriors of the past, who walked the razor's edge between life and death in the service of their king, meditated before battle, we too, as modern day warriors can vanquish the dangers of anticipation by cultivating a clear and tranquil mind. However, there are many types of meditation. Which is appropriate to achieve the result we as martial artists desire? One approach, as a preface to self-defense training, consists of sitting cross-legged in the half-lotus posture on a folded blanket to promote comfort (Figure 4-1). The hands are positioned in a gesture known as a *mudra*. *Mudra*, literally translated from Sanskrit, means "to seal". Thus the *mudra* is utilized to seal in the internal energy known as *Ki* which shall be examined in the next chapter. There are varieties of *mudras*, each symbolizing and meant to support a spiritual concept. The cosmic *mudra*, where the back of the left hand is placed in the palm of the right hand (reverse for women), thumbs touching, is a simple yet effective *mudra* to begin with (Figure 4-2). Make a perfect oval rather than permitting the thumbs to

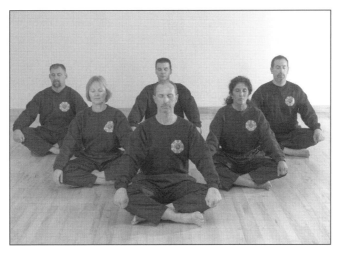

Figure 4-1

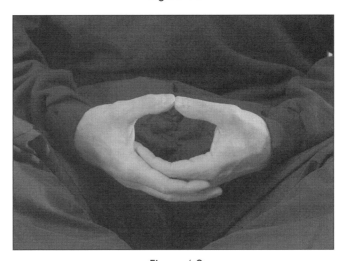

Figure 4-2

create a "peak" or the palms to collapse into a "valley." Let the hands rest gently in the lap, close the eyes and sit erect with the nose in line with the navel (Figure 4-3). Aside from allowing for a smooth exchange of breath, this posture encourages a free flow of *Ki*, or internal energy, to circulate throughout the body.

Using the breath as a focal point, slowly inhale through the nose and exhale through the mouth while assigning a single count to each cycle. Count to ten only and then return to one. Invariably, as you meditate, stray thoughts will attempt to invade the mind. Briefly acknowledge these feelings and permit them to pass through

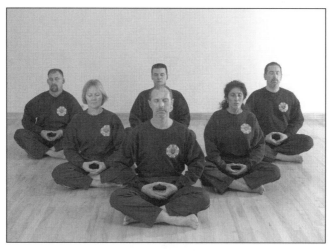

Figure 4-3

your consciousness, as would a gentle breeze, all the while returning to your breathing. Eventually, with patience and time, you may be able to abandon your counting altogether and simply focus on the breath. This basic method of meditation should serve to calm the mind prior to training and partially eliminate the distraction of anticipating a false technique rather than reacting to an intentional strike.

Moreover, as mentioned previously, enhancing the flow of *Ki* throughout the body is yet another objective of meditation. Why is this seemingly abstract action important to the martial artist? The manipulation of *Ki,* the universal life force, can be used for both benign and punitive purposes. For instance, in order to promote health, the practitioner of *kiatsu*, or *Ki* therapy, applies massage to the various acupoints that cover the body in an effort to stimulate a flow of *Ki*. When an abundant supply of *Ki* is present, a sense of well being pervades; when it is deficient, illness reigns. Likewise, the practice of acupuncture subscribes to the same principle by inserting needles at key points throughout the body to remove blockages in the series of pathways or meridians that traverse the human anatomy. The taekwondoist, on the other hand, channels *Ki* to a specific part of the body with the hope of projecting it through the striking surface whether it is a fist or a foot. This projection of *Ki* has the potential of amplifying the effectiveness of any technique many fold. *Ki* channeling can also be used to fortify the body at specific points thus preventing injury to the defender.

Naturally, these skills require long practice, but can be addressed through meditation and breathing exercises. While inhaling and exhaling, place your hands on your abdomen. What do you feel? When you inhale, the abdominal area should expand outward; by the same token, when you exhale, the same area should contract. This process is commonly known as normal or Buddhist breathing. Now, make a conscious effort to reverse this sequence, allowing the opposite to occur where the area surrounding your *tanjun*, or *Ki* center, two inches below the navel, contracts during inhalation and conversely expands when you exhale. This style of breathing is referred to as reverse or Taoist breathing, and represents an ancient method by which the respiratory process acts as a pump to move the flow of *Ki* through the meridians.

Sitting in the meditative posture described above, and employing the Taoist breathing method, visualize taking in a fresh, clean stream of *Ki* through the nose as you inhale and releasing a cloud of dark, used *Ki* similar to smoke, as you exhale. Following this meditation exercise, the body should feel revitalized and ready for vigorous practice. At some point, you can imagine lifting the *Ki* from the *tanjun* and mentally transporting it to various parts of the body. As a cautionary note, Taoist breathing can have ill effects if used excessively and should only be practiced for short periods of time.

Once, while training at the Korean National University for Physical Education in Seoul, South Korea, I was exposed to a radically different form of meditative motion that is intended to act as a bridge between the static, seated meditation depicted above, and the formal warm up routine. Best described as dynamic meditation, this exercise, taught to me by Master Jang Ki Park, is composed of a series of bends and stretches conjoined with focused breathing that is executed while seated in a half-lotus position. This meditative exercise, detailed photographically in my

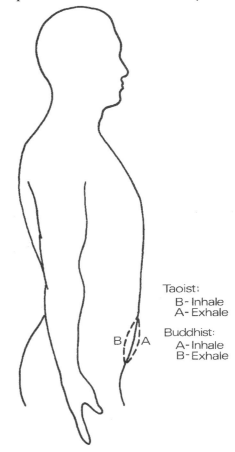

Taoist:
B - Inhale
A - Exhale

Buddhist:
A - Inhale
B - Exhale

Buddhist and Taoist Breathing.

book, *Taekwondo: Ancient Wisdom for the Modern Warrior,* published by YMAA Publication Center, serves to prepare the musculature and skeletal structure for the demands of flexibility training while igniting Ki through deep breathing.

CHAPTER 5

The Development and Use of Combat Ki

KI AND ITS NATURE

The practice of traditional taekwondo requires the student to become proficient in a multitude of blocks, kicks, strikes, and sweeps. However, in order to support these techniques far beyond the limitations of the physical body, one must introduce an element not easily definable in common terms. This element is referred to as *Ki* in Korean and *Qi* or *Chi* in Chinese.

Grandmaster Richard Chun, a true pioneer and practitioner of traditional taekwondo states that, "*Ki* is the cosmic ocean in which everything exists." Likewise, William Reed, a disciple of Koichi Tohei, founder of Shin Shin Totsu aikido, describes *Ki* as, "a universal energy capable of infinite expansion and contraction, which can be directed, but not contained, by the mind." In his book *Essential Anatomy*, hapkido practitioner Marc Tedeschi writes, "*Ki,* the vital life force, permeates the Universe, flowing through and animating all things."

Ki development is an essential component of martial arts training that is often overlooked in all likelihood due to the metaphysical issues it raises. Nevertheless,

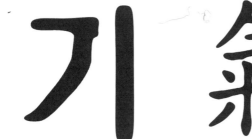

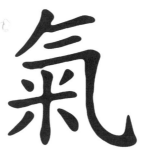

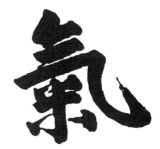

Hangul character for Ki.   Chinese character for Qi.   Japanese character for Ki.

teaching traditional taekwondo without offering the practitioner exercises in *Ki* development is tantamount to sitting someone behind the steering wheel of a car, but telling them nothing of the fuel that powers its engine. *Ki* is the elixir that amplifies technique and triggers great strength. It is the force that shields the body from harm while maintaining health and a sense of well being.

For centuries, since the publication of the *Nei Jing Su Wen*, or the *Classic on Internal Medicine*, by the Yellow Emperor, Huang Di (2697-2597 BC), Asian culture and Traditional Chinese Medicine in particular has recognized the existence of a force within the human body essential to the maintenance of life.

Today, the relevance of *Ki* is appreciated by millions of people who practice the disci-

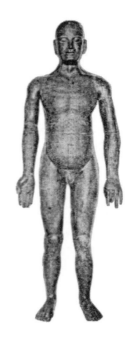

Bronze Man.

pline of *taijiquan*, benefit from the flowing postures unique to *qigong*, and find relief from pain through the treatment of acupuncture. Each of these arts in their own way relies on some form of *Ki* manipulation. Besides the martial arts, use of *Ki* is common to other disciplines unique to Asian culture: calligraphy, the tea ceremony, and flower arrangement, all rely on some form of *Ki* management in order to advance their practice. The structure of this vital life force still remains a mystery in no small part due to its evanescent nature. Studies have been conducted in an attempt to confirm the reality of *Ki* but at present, even though energy fields surrounding the body have been measured, no concrete clinical evidence is available to support its existence.

It is thought that several types of *Ki* dwelling in the body are represented by three physical states of matter. Michael Tse points out in his book, *QiGong for Health and Vitality*, that the universal life force first enters the body through the lungs intermingled with the air we breathe; thus the importance of deep, expansive breathing. Following extended practice, it is converted to liquid form and enters the circulatory system, revitalizing and cleansing the blood. Last and perhaps most intriguing, *Ki*, in its final stage of development solidifies, transforming into a crystalline structure with immense religious impact. Indeed, it is said that when enlightened beings of the

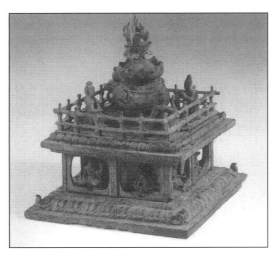

Sillian Reliquary.

Buddhist or Taoist faith perish, crystal beads are often discovered in the ashes that remain following the cremation of the human form. This coveted substance is called *xie li zi* (or *sarira* in Korean) and, once collected, is deposited in metallic reliquaries that are safely stored in stone pagodas within temple walls. Once, while traveling in Korea, our group visited Bulguksa Temple in Kyongju where this fact, much to my satisfaction, was confirmed by our temple guide.

Nevertheless, as martial artists looking to support technique, it is the rich mixture of *Ki* and air that we are most concerned with. Because this ether maintains a constant link with the universe, our body can be considered a vessel through which the vital life force maintains a spiritual connection between heaven and the earth. *Ki*, in this sense then is borrowed, constantly re-circulated, but never owned. It is benevolent in nature and, therefore, cannot be abused or put to use frivolously. If called upon with false motives or arrogant intent, it will fail every time.

Physically, *Ki* can be thought of as a bioelectric current. Subsequently, the martial artist can use this energy to "short circuit" another's malevolent energy causing it to betray him in the process. One basis for this assumption is that everything in nature is composed of matter vibrating at different energy levels; molecules are composed of atoms bound together by electrons orbiting a minute nucleus, all with negative and positive charges. If the practitioner can cause his adversary's kinetic energy to flicker, even for a moment through the use of *Ki* manipulation, then he has gained the upper hand even before a blow has been dealt. Again, while this effect, defined as combat *Ki,* is unsubstantiated by science, it stands as the cornerstone of many classical martial disciplines such as hapkido and aikido that rely on yielding to an opponent's negative intentions.

THE MERIDIANS

To understand *Ki* and its movement through the body, it is helpful to visualize systems in nature with which we are familiar. In doing so, both the human circulatory system and an ordinary electrical circuit come to mind. Both rely on a physical pathway for transportation. Arteries, veins, and capillaries carry blood. Copper wire transports electricity. What, then, conveys *Ki*? *Ki* is thought to travel through a series of channels or meridians that span the body. The two grand meridians, located on the front and back of the torso, feed a complimentary series of channels. These pathways known as the twelve regular meridians are associated with specific organs of the body as follows: lung, large intestine, stomach, spleen, heart, small intestine, bladder, kidney, pericardium, Triple Warmer, gall bladder, and liver. An additional eight, grouped in pairs, are known as the extraordinary meridians, and perform a separate function.

Nevertheless, all of these meridians are invisible to the eye resulting in great skepticism concerning their existence. However, it is these very meridians and their related pressure points that the acupuncturist stimulates for therapeutic purposes and the martial artist activates to support technique. By removing blockages in the meridian system, which can cause illness and in extreme cases, death, the practitioner of Traditional Chinese Medicine has the power to cure a variety of diseases. Conversely, the taekwondoist, by striking one or more of the many acupoints that dot the body, can incapacitate an attacker. Metaphorically speaking, these pressure points are similar to stations along a railway. Yet, rather than bearing the name of a town or village, they are designated by a number and the anatomical organ with which they are associated. The meridians mirror the tracks while *Ki* itself would be the engine traveling along the rails. While this analogy is simplistic at best, it crudely describes the method of how *Ki* is distributed throughout the body.

THE TANJUN

Located two inches below the navel, the *tanjun* in Korean or *dantien* in Chinese, represents the reservoir from which *Ki* radiates. In Chinese, *dan* is defined as crystal or the essence of energy, while *tien* is translated as the area for the essence of energy. It is here that *Ki* is stored after entering the body. According to Reed, the *tanjun* is best described as the "one-point, a tiny star, or vortex sucking in immense amounts of energy from the universe."

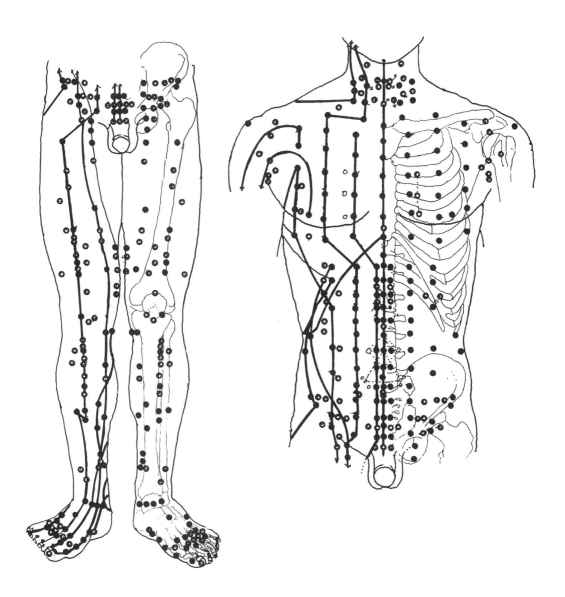

Primary Meridians and acupuncture cavities on the front of the body.

There are many theories regarding the *tanjun*, the foremost being that it is the physical, cellular center of the human anatomy from which the body develops outward from conception. It is also considered one's natural center of gravity around which the extremities move. This concept becomes all the more evident when we view the contrasting outlooks between Eastern and Western culture in regards to the hub of human intent. In Western society, we often say that we "think from the heart"; heartache, heartbreak, and heart-felt thanks are all conceptual indicators of this principle. Conversely, in Eastern thought, intention is said to emanate from the *hara* (in Japanese) or, as we now know in Korean, the *tanjun*. This fundamental difference in belief reflects the conviction that the vital life force is distributed from the body's center and, thus, can be stored, channeled, manipulated, and amplified to promote health and intensify technique in the case of the martial artist. Hence, it can be said that *Ki* not only projects, but also protects.

PRACTICES CULTIVATING THE KI FLOW

Yet, before one can knowingly utilize *Ki* to their advantage, they must first acknowledge and trust in its existence. This requires a leap of faith for many Westerners. Accepting this, however, there are a number of exercises that can be practiced to cultivate *Ki* flow and focus. One such exercise, taught to me by my instructor Grandmaster Richard Chun in preparation for black belt class, finds two students facing one another, seated in horse stance (Figure 5-1). Students A and B then lock their right and left wrists together respectively forming ridge hands in a palm up position (Figure 5-2). Notice that the inactive hand is chambered at the hip. Tensing the *tanjun* and upper body, A and B then alternate pushing and resisting as the hands describe a crescent motion inward and outward relative to the body (Figure 5-3). The breath must be synchronized by inhaling before beginning the crescent motion and then exhaling as the movement is executed. After five repetitions, the placement of the ridge hand should be switched to accommodate practice with both the inner and outer edge of the wrists and hands (Figure 5-4). Both students then reverse sides

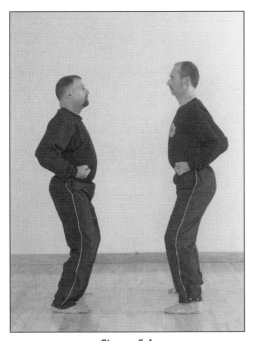

Figure 5-1

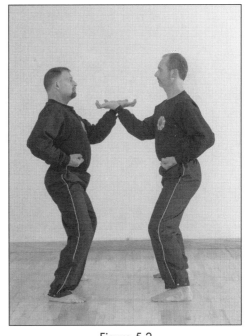

Figure 5-2

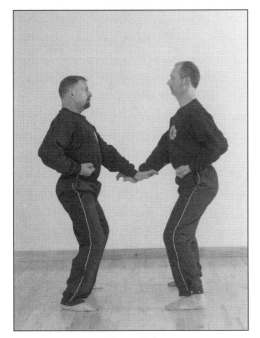

Figure 5-3

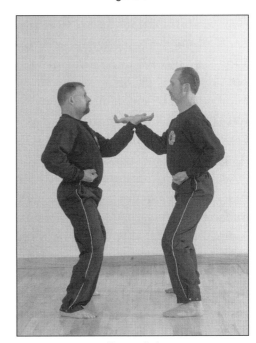

Figure 5-4

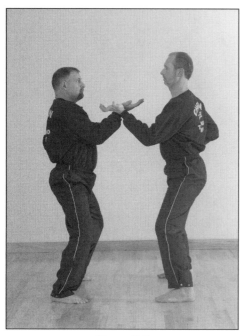

Figure 5-5

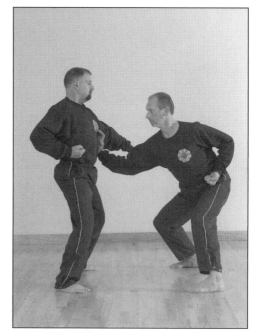

Figure 5-6

(Figure 5-5). During this exercise, the student visualizes the *Ki* flowing upward from *tanjun* through the meridians, eventually finding its way to the blade edge of the ridge hand. The successful execution of this technique not only strengthens the upper body, but also begins to teach the practitioner how to draw *Ki* to a blocking surface. This sequence can be supplemented by adding a controlled palm heel strike to the partner's solar plexus following the downward crescent motion of the ridge hand (Figure 5-6). Correctly done, student B should sense a penetrating energy extending from student A's palm.

Once the *Ki* has been stimulated through the above practice, the martial artist can advance to an exercise that resembles a game, yet in reality is intended to enhance one's ability to sense an opponent's energy and act upon it. Starting out in a front stance (*ap koobi*), student A and student B place the outer edges of their lead foot together (Figure 5-7). Next, they clasp lead hands as if in greeting (Figure 5-8). The object of this exercise is to break your partner's balance by yielding to, and then redirecting, the advance of their negative *Ki* (Figure 5-9). Invariably, A, or B, will attempt to disrupt their partner's stability by either pushing or pulling haphazardly. When this occurs, the opposite partner, sensing aggressive *Ki*, will yield to the uncontrolled, negative movement, thus causing their partner to falter.

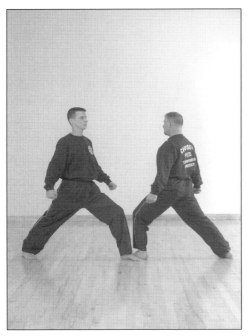

Figure 5-7

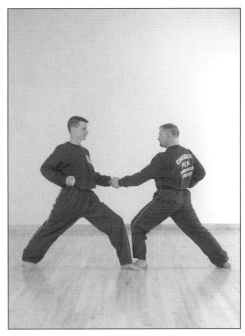

Figure 5-8

BREATHING TO CULTIVATE KI FLOW

Since it has been determined that deep breathing is the primary method of capturing *Ki* from the universe, exercises that promote the inhalation and exhalation of air are strongly recommended. One needs only consider the calming effect a deep breath has on an anxious individual to appreciate the advantage of this action. Couple this technique with a visualization tool that stimulates *Ki* flow through the

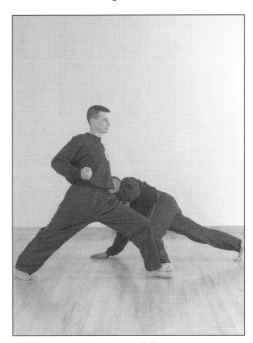

Figure 5-9

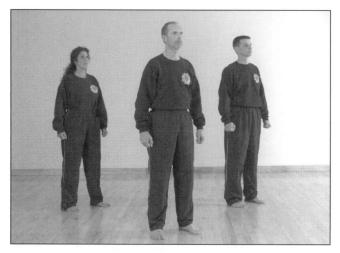

Figure 5-10

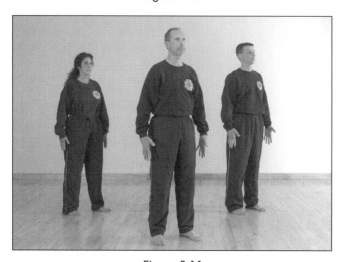

Figure 5-11

meridians, and you are left with a powerful and comprehensive *Ki* development exercise that promotes deep *tanjun* breathing. First, stand upright with the feet shoulder width apart (Figure 5-10). Next, splay the fingers wide, palms facing each other (Figure 5-11). Close the eyes and inhale deeply through the nose, feeling a connection with the universe. Be mindful of the *Ki* traveling internally down the front of the body, through the meridians, until it reaches the *tanjun*. Simultaneously, bend

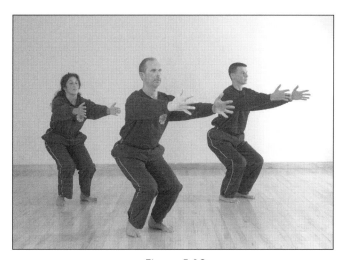

Figure 5-12

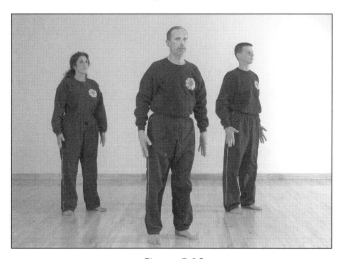

Figure 5-13

the knees while extending the arms forward (Figure 5-12). At this point, the practitioner should take a moment to sense the *Ki* coursing through the body, emanating from the *tanjun*, traversing the meridians in the torso and, subsequently, extending to the extremities. Visualize the energy shooting out of the fingertips and rooting you to the earth through the soles of the feet. Lastly, exhale through the mouth and straighten the body, bringing the hands back to your sides (Figure 5-13).

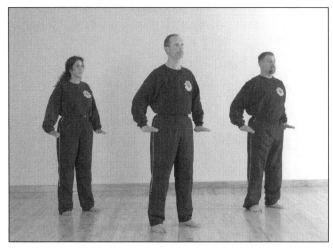

Figure 5-14

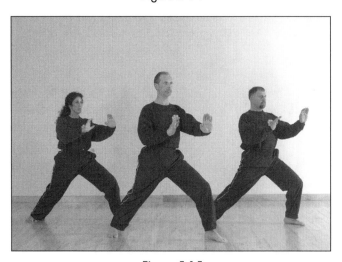

Figure 5-15

DYNAMIC EXERCISES

Aside from the static exercises just described, there are a number of dynamic, moving exercises that can be performed to enhance the flow of *Ki* without the use of a partner. One particular sequence, known as the Boulder Push, requires the student to stand upright with both palms facing the floor (Figure 5-14). While maintaining this transitory position, the student inhales deeply through the nose and then strongly exhales through the mouth while stepping with the left leg into an extended front stance (*ap koobi*). At the same time, the upper body is tensed and the hands slowly push forward,

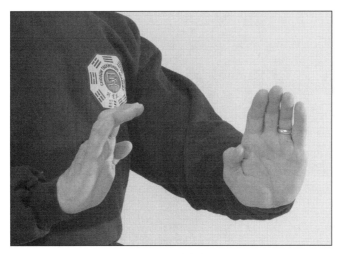

Figure 5-16

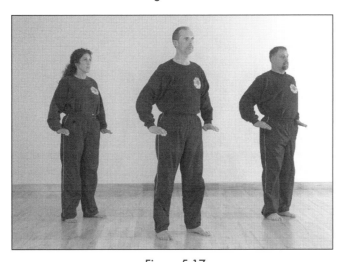

Figure 5-17

palms out, as if driving a great boulder away from the body (Figure 5-15). Notice that the left hand is slightly extended in relation to the right (Figure 5-16). The sequence continues with the student again assuming the upright, transitory stance, palms facing down (Figure 5-17). Stepping forward with the right leg, both hands push forward with the right slightly extended. The upper body again is tensed in synchronization with a strong exhalation of breath through the mouth (Figure 5-18).

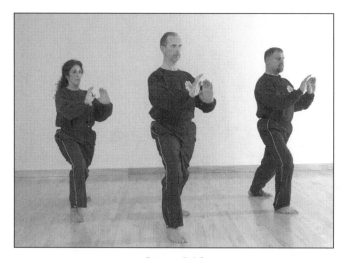

Figure 5-18

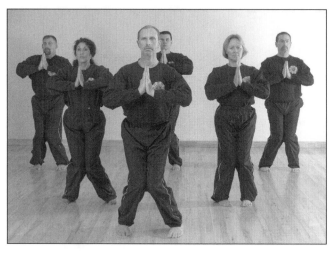

Figure 5-19

In doing research for this work, I came across a highly effective *Ki* development exercise used by practitioners of *kumdo*, or "the Way of the Korean sword," to enhance *Ki* circulation, balance, strength, and extension of the vital life force. This exercise also represents a form of *tanjun ho hup*, or deep *Ki* breathing. Such is the value of this method that it has become a staple of our training regimen.

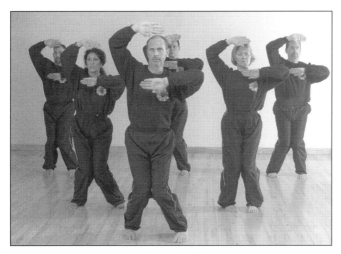

Figure 5-20

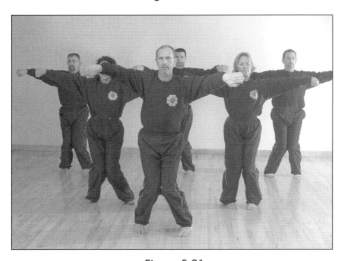

Figure 5-21

Dropping into a modified horse stance with both knees touching, the martial artist presses the palms together, fingertips pointed upward, to promote *Ki* circulation through the *lao gong*, an acupoint situated in the center of the palm claimed to be the most sensitive area of the body for *Ki* projection (Figure 5-19). Next, the right hand is placed above the left, palms facing outward with the practitioner gazing between both (Figure 5-20). This motion mimics the *Um/Yang* and cultivates balance. With the fingers hooking in towards the palms, the hands are then drawn back towards the body and down (Figure 5-21). At hip level, fists are made and lifted to

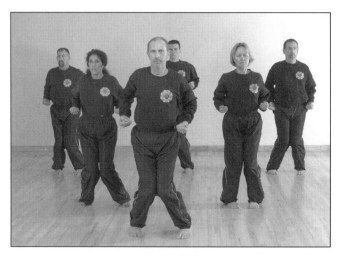

Figure 5-22

the armpits in an isometric exercise to develop upper body strength (Figure 5-22). Finally, the hands are once again opened and execute *momtang milgi makki* or pushing middle block (Figure 5-23). The goal of this technique is to extend *Ki* outward from the *lao gong*. A similar set of dynamic motions can be practiced in a seated position as well. Practiced diligently over time, strength and muscle tone can be dramatically increased.

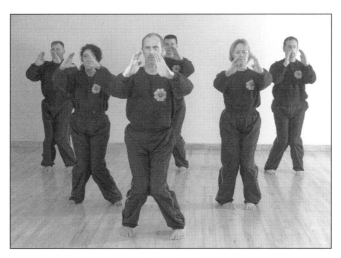

Figure 5-23

It is important to remember that there are no winners or losers in Ki development exercises; they are not shows of strength or a demonstration of one's power over another. Each movement in solo performance or between partners must be done with sincerity and cooperation if any benefit is to be gained. Ki is benevolent in nature and, therefore refuses to be abused. Through it, the martial artist can dominate, but not terrorize. If the practitioner of qigong, acupuncture, or the martial arts attempts to manipulate Ki for selfish or malevolent purposes other than cultural tradition, therapeutic value, or self-defense, it is sure to fail them every time. Called upon properly, however, with respect, dignity, and benign intent, it will focus intention, heal, nurture a sense of well being, and support taekwondo technique far beyond the limitations of the physical self.

CHAPTER 6
The Relevance of Poom-Se
in Traditional Taekwondo

Forms can be defined as choreographed sequences of techniques aimed at defeating multiple attackers advancing from various directions. Characterized in Korean as *poom-se*, *hyung*, *tul*, in Chinese as *kuen*, and in Japanese as *kata*, forms represent the essence of any classical martial art. Over the centuries, prior to the advent of sport sparring, forms practice constituted the primary means by which effective self-defense strategy was recorded and transmitted from venerable master to disciple, elder to warrior. Recognizing that *poom-se* represents a significant portion of the traditional taekwondo curriculum, Grandmaster Richard Chun, in the first edition of his landmark book, *Advancing in Taekwondo*, remarks "without forms there is no taekwondo." This notion is echoed by many who view *poom-se* training as a valuable tool in building defensive skills.

With the recognition of the influence foreign nations have had on the growth of the Korean martial arts, the origin of taekwondo *poom-se* can be traced back centuries to the year 1377 AD when an alliance was forged between China and Okinawa that

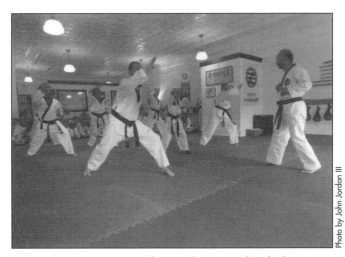

Poom-Se practice with Grandmaster Richard Chun.

resulted in a great infusion of Chinese culture. In 1429, the immigration of Chinese nationals adept in the art of *kempo* greatly influenced the native combative styles of the island kingdom. The towns of Shuri and Naha, bolstered by this expansion in trade, would come to be known for the combative systems that they would eventually spawn. Many of the *kata* practiced in karate today such as *Kushanku* and *Wanshu,* still bear the names of the Chinese practitioners who inspired them. Then, as Okinawa moved from a provincial to a regional economy, relations were established between Indonesia, Japan, and Korea.

During the latter part of the fifteenth century, an event occurred that would have a pronounced effect on the practice of empty-hand self-defense. King Sho Shin of

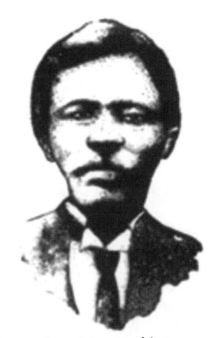

Yasutsune Itosu. Originator of the Pinan Kata.

Okinawa forbade the ownership of weapons by civilians and required that all nobles relocate to within the shadow of Shuri Castle. This prohibition caused the citizens to find alternative methods of self-protection and since combat skill was rewarded by the king, many in the nobility practiced empty-hand martial arts.

Following the successful invasion of Okinawa by Japan in 1609, forms, or martial arts patterns, took on additional importance. Driven by a continued ban on arms, the citizenry had learned to employ farm and household items as weapons. Oars, pitchforks, and scythes, that would later evolve into specialized martial arts weapons, found their way into the secretive practice of *kata.*

Japan in 1868 began to democratize its society and transition from feudalism to a system of democracy. In the process, much in the way of tradition was obfuscated with the exception of martial arts training, transformed instead from a necessary component of military combat to a vehicle for promoting morality, health, and fitness. Suddenly the native defensive arts, devoid of their battlefield tactics, took on the complexion of sports-oriented pursuits.

With efforts beginning in 1901, Yasutsune Itosu, ushered in the twentieth century by introducing karate into the Okinawan school system with the goal of cultivating physical fitness and a strong character in children.

This was primarily accomplished through the use of "sanitized" *kata*. Since, at least for the children, self-defense was not the main focus of instruction, the practical applications of techniques within the form were intentionally masked in ambiguity. This method of teaching represented a major shift in forms training that would have ramifications far into the future. Criticized for diluting the fundamental purpose of *kata*, and thus karate in general since forms remained the essence of the art, Itosu later wrote, "You must decide whether your *kata* is for cultivation of health or for its practical use." He further advised adult students to, "Always practice *kata* with its practical use in mind."

The historical perspective submitted earlier in this book now begins to take on an added dimension since we now start to see

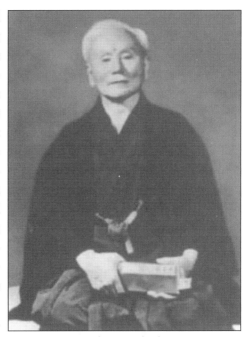

Gichin Funakoshi.

how *poom-se* that are today unique to the Korean martial arts were influenced by events that occurred in neighboring countries shortly before, or concurrent with, the Japanese Occupation of the nation from 1910 to 1945. Clearly, the practice of karate required a deep understanding and respect for *kata* that continues to stand as a centerpiece for its practice to this day. This principle must surely have been inculcated in the minds of Won Kuk Lee and General Choi, Hong Hi while studying in Japan under the direction of Gichin Funakoshi, founder of Shotokan Karate-Do.

If memory serves, both of these innovators, soon to promote the martial arts within the borders of their native land, returned home from abroad undoubtedly with practical knowledge of the *Shotokan Heian, Pinan, Bassai,* and *Tekki kata* that would ultimately evolve into the *Kicho, Pyung-An, Balsek,* and *Chul-Ki poom-se* of *tae soo do,* and later, taekwondo. Therefore, it is fair to conclude that many of the forms performed during the evolutionary years of traditional taekwondo mirrored the *kata* of Shotokan karate. A close look at Funakoshi's work, *Karate-Do Kyohan,* first published in 1936, confirms this fact when one compares the movements of *Tekki Shodan* to that of *Chul-Ki Cho Dan.*

In founding his style of taekwondo, General Choi, Hong Hi paved the way for the future by developing the *Chang-Han* set of formal exercises that bore the shadow of techniques culled from his training in karate-do. A quote from his fifteen-volume, *Encyclopedia of Taekwondo*, first issued in 1983, delineates the important position forms training holds in the traditional taekwondo curriculum by stating that, "Though sparring may merely indicate that an opponent is more or less advanced, patterns are a more critical barometer in evaluating an individual's technique."

The *Chang-Han* series of ITF forms currently consist of twenty-four patterns and differ significantly from others in the fact that their movements subscribe to a "wave" or "sign-curve" motion of the body as it transitions from sequence to sequence. This unique dynamic is believed to dramatically amplify power to blocks and strikes. Moreover, the *kihop*, or spirit yell, uttered forcefully as a means of punctuating specific strikes and kicks found in forms of other styles, have been eliminated favoring instead equal power on every technique.

PALGWE, TAEGEUK, AND BLACK BELT POOM-SE SERIES

Following General Choi's exodus from Korea and the eventual establishment of the World Taekwondo Federation (WTF) by a younger generation of practitioners not directly affected by Japanese instruction, two new sets of forms were developed in an effort to eliminate any vestige of Japanese influence. The elder *Palgwe* series came into existence during the early 1970s and were intended to test the proficiency of color belt, or *gup* level, students. The overriding concept of these patterns derives from the *Palgwe*: a Taoist symbol depicting a central *Yin/Yang* surrounded by eight trigrams.

These forms tend to emphasize lower stances coupled with a variety of effective hand techniques. Taken as a complete set, the eight *Palgwe poom-se* share a philosophical underpinning similar to those of their more recent kin, the *Taegeuk* series.

As taekwondo began to evolve into a combat sport with Olympic aspirations, a method was required to teach and support the upright fighting stance used in competition. Originally intended to replace the *Palgwe*, the eight *poom-se* of the *Taegeuk* set feature the walking, or natural stance (*ap sogi*) in many sequences; a posture not seen in earlier forms. If viewed from above, the pattern of movements within the forms trace the Chinese symbol for "king." Bearing the namesake of the Korean flag, the *Taegeuk* patterns were created in the late 1970s with, as we shall see, philosophical principles running parallel to those of the *Palgwe* series.

Once the student reaches black belt level, a more demanding set of *poom-se* are introduced with roots that date back to the mid 1960s. Developed by the Korea Taekwondo Association, and later refined and sanctioned by the World Taekwondo Federation, the nine WTF Black Belt *poom-se* follow lines of motion described by

Taekwondo Poom-Se: Palgwe Ee Jang
☰ *Philosophy: Lake* ☱

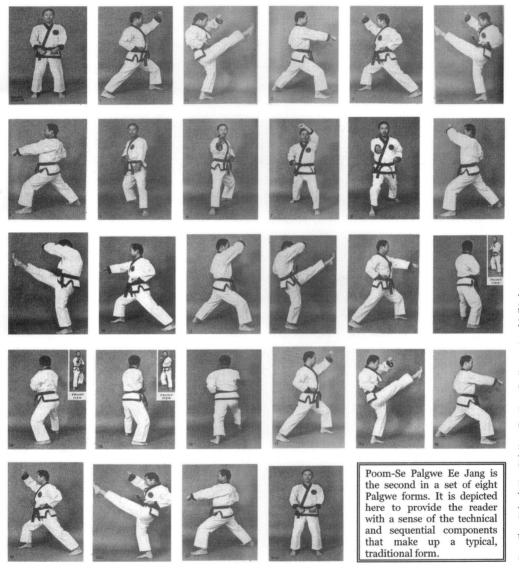

Poom-Se Palgwe Ee Jang is the second in a set of eight Palgwe forms. It is depicted here to provide the reader with a sense of the technical and sequential components that make up a typical, traditional form.

From Chun, Richard. *Moo Duk Kwan Tae Kwon Do Korean Art of Self-Defense* Santa Clarita: Ohara Publications, 1975.

A taekwondo poom-se can be defined as a sequence of choreographed techniques aimed at defeating multiple opponents attacking from different directions. It is the method by which native Korean martial arts skills were transmitted from venerable master to disciple over the decades. Each has a unique philosophy attached to it.

Poom-Se Palgwe Ee Jang.

Chinese and Korean characters that depict the underlying philosophy of the *poom-se*. These patterns contain advanced techniques unique to the dan grade holder.

Besides the *hyung*, or *poom-se*, mentioned above, other forms exist that are unique to differing styles of taekwondo. For instance, members of *Moo Duk Kwan* Taekwondo, or the Institute of Martial Virtue, one of the primordial *kwans* previously visited in our historical retrospective, practice *Sip Soo*, and *Jion*; forms that claim Chinese ancestry. Likewise, the *Pyung-Ahn* set consisting of five *hyung*, continue to be practiced by those *dojangs* with a deep respect for tradition. Furthermore, although taekwondo is primarily an empty-hand art, often sword (*jook-do*) and fighting staff (*jong bong*) forms are added to the curriculum at advanced levels.

Each *poom-se*, *hyung*, or *tul*, whether it is of WTF or ITF pedigree, contains a series of blocks, kicks, and strikes executed through a range of stances across a predetermined pattern. The sequence and intricacy of the individual techniques determines the complexity of the form and, therefore, the level at which it is taught. By way of example, *Kicho Ilbo*, the first form in a set of three reserved for the beginner, includes one block followed by a strike, performed in front stance (*ap koobi*). In contrast, *Palgwe Pal Jang*, the last in a series of eight, is significantly more complex requiring additional expertise on the part of the maturing martial artist.

Individual forms that appear in groups, especially those found in the *Taegeuk*, *Palgwe* or *Chul-Ki* series, can be viewed as single volumes within an encyclopedia, or the chapters of a book, each containing a unique combination of techniques not found elsewhere. In fact, the suffix *Jang* that follows the number of the form in either the *Palgwe* or *Taegeuk* set can be translated from the Korean as "chapter." Subsequently, it is not unusual for the black belt student to practice *poom-se* aimed specifically to the novice in the hope of growing ever closer to the core of the combined techniques. Indeed, with each successive performance the diligent practitioner moves from one level of proficiency to the next, from the physical to the meditative.

Aside from developing one's ability to defend and counterattack, *poom-se* training offers many ancillary benefits. However, given the fact that the primary goal of forms training is the inculcation of defensive skills, these often go unnoticed until they are appreciated in retrospect. For instance, balance is enhanced by virtue of the dynamic footwork required to segue from stance to stance. The necessity of responding rapidly to directional changes develops agility. Likewise, the synchronization of breath to motion fortifies the body with a fresh supply of *Ki* while supporting technique. Through this synergy, the muscles enjoy a relaxed state causing speed to manifest as power. This principle is all the more important since taekwondo, as we have seen, is an amalgam of both hard and soft martial arts styles with roots in Japanese karate and Chinese gungfu. Furthermore, a great sense of achievement is realized when the student finally rises above the struggle of learning to perform a particular *poom-se* in the first place.

To the casual onlooker, it is easy to confuse the performance of *poom-se* visually with that of modern dance. In fact, as Grandmaster Sang Kyu Shim points out in his inspirational book, *The Making of a Martial Artist*, the taekwondoist is more akin to a dancer than a boxer. Nevertheless, make no mistake, for while this analogy suggests the poise and grace common to physically artistic pursuits such as dance, this is where the similarity ends. If practiced diligently with purpose and focused intent, coupled with a working knowledge of the sequenced techniques involved, *poom-se* practice can cultivate articulate self-defense skills executed in rapid-fire fashion.

LEARNING POOM-SE

The process of learning and internalizing *poom-se* can be divided into various categories and sub-categories. The first stage is what we shall refer to as *Technique to Count*. This is where the form is broken down into its individual components and executed by numbered count. While robotic in appearance, this method allows the practitioner to refine each block, kick, or strike before stringing them together in a cohesive pattern. Gross motions are taught first leaving the distillation of detail for later. Only a small portion of the form should be transmitted within a given training session allowing the mind and body to become acquainted with transition as well as technique. At this point, there is little thought given to the philosophical underpinning of the *poom-se* still to come.

Once the entire form has been memorized and can be performed flawlessly to count, the sequences that define its defensive structure are introduced. Suddenly, the *poom-se* begins to come alive and manifest its true protective nature; single techniques combine to reveal interrelated packets of defensive strategy. This portion of the *poom-se* learning curve, referred to as *Sequence to Count*, reflects an ever deepening understanding of the form.

Once both the individual count and sequenced count approach is perfected, *Physical Practice* follows with the taekwondoist executing the *poom-se* with fluidity, strength, and focus while vigorously imitating a response to an authentic self-defense scenario. Concurrently, breath control, with each inhalation and exhalation being synchronized to motion, is practiced. Moreover, as the maturing martial artist grows to appreciate the value and potential power of the universal life force, *Ki* will be projected to punctuate technique and penetrate the imaginary target. If performed correctly, vigorous forms practice can offer an aerobic benefit similar to that of a well-fought sparring match and is certain to have a pronounced effect on stamina. The *Physical Practice* stage requires great patience since hundreds of repetitions must be performed before the practitioner can truly claim the *poom-se* as their own.

The final and the least understood phase of forms training is *Meditative Practice* centering on the philosophical principles that underscore traditional *poom-se*. In this, the most challenging and transcendental stage of *poom-se* training, the practitioner begins to dwell on the meaning and lessons that highlight a given form. Invariably, one may ask, why does something as apparently violent as a choreographed sequence of martial arts techniques need to mirror philosophical doctrine? Moreover, why should the practice of a modern Olympic sport be distracted by a system of esoteric principles based on Taoist thought? And lastly, how is it possible for a series of martial exercises that were created in the latter part of the twentieth century to reflect an ancient ideology?

MORAL DEVELOPMENT IN TAEKWONDO PRACTICE

The truth is that any classical martial discipline worthy of its holistic intent needs to be governed by a set of moral safeguards that limit its use. Furthermore, a prime objective of martial arts training in the twenty-first century is the enhancement of mind, body, and spirit through disciplined practice thus lending credence to the time-tested philosophical principles that surround forms. On a competitive level, while at first glance these ideals may seem outdated as they relate to the modern combat sport of taekwondo, they in fact are all the more relevant when viewed as a blueprint for virtuous behavior at ringside by many contestants.

Admittedly, the conveyance of virtue espoused in traditional taekwondo is often confusing, appearing both obvious and mystical at the same time. For instance, most practitioners are taught the Five Tenets including courtesy, integrity, perseverance, self-control, and indomitable spirit early in their training and steered by an ethical compass that can be traced back to a set of directives handed down to the Hwarang warriors in seventh-century Silla by the Buddhist monk, Wonkwang Popsa. However, deeper still lies another, less evident spring of knowledge that flows from the philosophical principles that amplify both WTF *poom-se* and ITF *tul*. To fully grasp this concept, the taekwondoist must first be taught and accept that underlying each form is a specific philosophy that can easily be applied to situations that arise in everyday life. It is imperative, however, that practitioners first appreciate the source from which these philosophical doctrines derive.

It is said that almost five thousand years ago, a Taoist sage by the name of Fu Hsi (2953-2838 BCE) composed the *I Ching*, or *The Book of Changes*, considered by many

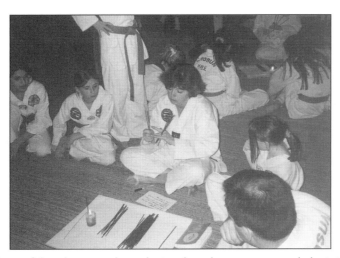

Students of the Chosun Taekwondo Academy learning to consult the I Ching.

to be a cornerstone of Taoist philosophy. This classic, later amended by Confucius, acted as an oracle for those seeking advice in business, politics, military affairs, and life in general.

The formula for use of this compendium is based largely upon the duality of opposites or the *Yin/Yang* (*Um/Yang* in Korean). The *Yin/Yang* is surrounded by eight trigrams or *gwe* composed of solid and broken lines that subsequently combine to create sixty four hexagrams thus giving us the final tools necessary to manipulate the *I Ching*. If one were to examine the eight original trigrams, however, they would discover a direct correlation between their meanings and the philosophical components that lie behind the eight *Taegeuk* and *Palgwe poom-se* sanctioned by the WTF that we are familiar with today.

For instance, *Taegeuk Yook Jang*, whose *I Ching* component is a broken line over a solid line with another broken line beneath, symbolizes water and focuses on our ability to overcome life's hardships by exhibiting the consistency and flow of a great river. Likewise, *poom-se Taegeuk Chil Jang* is signified by two broken lines below a single, solid line. The philosophical principle of this *poom-se* is mountain and teaches the practitioner when to advance and when to hesitate, mirroring the behavior of an experienced climber as they progressively attain the summit. Additionally, all eight WTF Black Belt *poom-se* are steeped in traditional principles ranging from *Koryo*, a form demonstrating strength as expressed through conviction, to *poom-se Ilyo* representing the Buddhist spiritual quest for oneness or nirvana.

A discrete set of ideals, in many cases tied to personalities and events in Korean history are assigned to the ITF forms or tul, created by General Choi. By way of

(continued on page 79)

Poomse Philosophical Concepts
and their
Relationship to the Eight Trigrams of the I Ching

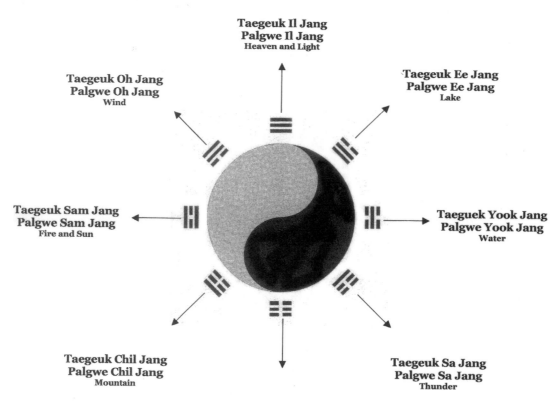

Taegeuk Il Jang
Palgwe Il Jang
Heaven and Light

Taegeuk Oh Jang
Palgwe Oh Jang
Wind

Taegeuk Ee Jang
Palgwe Ee Jang
Lake

Taegeuk Sam Jang
Palgwe Sam Jang
Fire and Sun

Taeguek Yook Jang
Palgwe Yook Jang
Water

Taegeuk Chil Jang
Palgwe Chil Jang
Mountain

Taegeuk Sa Jang
Palgwe Sa Jang
Thunder

Taegeuk Pal Jang
Palgwe Pal Jang
Earth

Taegeuk and Palgwe Poom-Se Philosophy

Poom-Se	I Ching Symbol	Concept	Philosophy
Taegeuk Il Jang Palgwe Il Jang		Keon	**Heaven and Light:** These elementary formal exercises represent the source of creation by presenting the most basic of techniques to the novice. They contain pure yang energy.
Taegeuk Ee Jang Palgwe Ee Jang		Tae	**Lake:** These forms represent a spiritually uplifting nature with a firm state of mind through which virtue smiles. Movements should be made in a relaxed manner yet with firm control.
Taegeuk Sam Jang Palgwe Sam Jang		Ri	**Fire and Sun:** These forms should be performed with the warmth and enthusiasm that accompanies the unpredictable pace and passion found in the flames of fire.
Taegeuk Sa Jang Palgwe Sa Jang		Jin	**Thunder:** Just as a fearsome thunderstorm passes leaving rain freshened air in its wake, these forms teach us to act bravely in the face of danger knowing it too shall pass.
Taegeuk Oh Jang Palgwe Oh Jang		Seon	**Wind:** Yielding but penetrating, soothing yet destructive, this, the fifth forms in the series must reflect the characteristics of a gentle summer breeze or a mighty hurricane.
Taegeuk Yook Jang Palgwe Yook Jang		Gam	**Water:** Just as water can wear down the hardest of rocks over time, these forms teach patience, consistency and flow. Humility, too, is refined since water always flows downward.
Taegeuk Chil Jang Palgwe Chil Jang		Gan	**Mountain:** Climbing a great mountain, one must develop the wisdom of when to hesitate and when to move ahead. The dual principles of stability and ambition are appreciated.
Taegeuk Pal Jang Palgwe Pal Jang		Gon	**Earth:** Receptive, gentle and nurturing, the Earth provides the substance into which the forces of creation pass. Checking all prior leaning, these forms contain pure um energy.

World Taekwondo Federation Black Belt Poom-Se Philosophy

Poom-Se	Concept	Philosophy
Koryo	Korea	The first poom-se of nine in the WTF black belt series memorializes the Koryo Dynasty and reflects the indomitable will expressed by the Korean people in the face of extreme adversity. The country name Korea derives from the word Koryo.
Keumgang	Diamond	Just as a diamond exhibits hardness, and beauty through clarity, this form must express the spiritual strength necessary to cut through all distractions presented by life. Named after the Keumgang-San mountain range, this form describes the Chinese character for mountain.
Taebaek	Mountain	In the year 2333 BC, the legendary Tan-Gun founded a nation in Taebaek on Mount Baekdoo. This form venerates this most sacred of mountains. Also, since this mountain reaches to the sun, Taebaek can be defined as "light" and must be performed with the agility of light.
Pyongwon	Plain	The unbroken expanse of a plain bestows a sense of majesty upon mankind while presenting an impression different from that one receives when viewing tall mountains or endless forests. This form must express the majestic but friendly spirit of a vast plain.
Sipjin	Decimal	Describing the Chinese character for ten, this form expresses endless development and growth, but a highly orderly and predictable growth that fosters stability. Therefore, each movement of this form must follow an orderly and systematic progression.
Jitae	Earth	The earth hides its greatest power deep within its fiery core, occasionally permitting it to well up and shake civilization, reminding mankind of his frailties. This form must show the vigor of life as it stems from the power welling up from strong muscles and a deep, powerful core.
Cheonkwon	Sky	This form must exhibit the piety and awe that the sky commands as well as the vitality it sparks in man's imagination, driving him to strive upward. Cheonkwon should demonstrate man's emotions as he looks up from earth and is reminded of an eagle flying off into the clouds.
Hansoo	Water	Like water, which is the source of life, the strength of taekwondo stems not from stubbornness and the refusal to yield but rather from fluidity and adaptability. This form epitomizes these qualities. Therefore, its forcefulness must originate from its fluidity.
Ilyo	Oneness	Stemming from Buddhism, the goal of spiritual life is Ilyo; oneness or nirvana. Only in this state is ego overcome. The ideal of taekwondo is Ilyo. It is a discipline in which you concentrate your attention on every movement and in doing so, shed all worldly thoughts and preconceptions.

International Taekwon-Do Federation Tul Philosophy

Tul	Philosophy
Chon-Ji	Literally translated as Heaven and Earth, this pattern consists of one section superimposed over the over, one representing Heaven, the other Earth. This form is intended for the beginning student.
Tan-Gun	This pattern immortalizes the legendary founder of Korea, Tan-Gun, who it is said established the Korean nation of Ko-Chosun in Taebaek among the mists of Mount Baekdoo in the year 2333 BC.
Do-San	Although its title is a pseudonym, this pattern pays tribute to the patriot Ahn Chang Ho (1876-1938) who actively worked for the Korean independence movement and to further educate the Korean people.
Won-Hyo	A highly influential personality in Korean history, Won-Hyo, meaning dawn, was responsible for introducing Buddhism to the Korean peninsula during the Silla Dynasty in the year 686 AD.
Yul-Gok	Nicknamed the "Confucius of Korea", this form memorializes the great philosopher Yi I (1536-1584). The *tul's* pattern of movement traces the character for the word "scholar".
Joong-Gun	Named after the patriot Ahn Joong Gun for his role in the assassination of Hirobumi Ito, the first Japanese resident-general, this pattern consists of 32 movements that represent Ahn's age at his execution.
Toi-Gye	This pattern venerates the noted scholar and authority on Neo-Confucianism, Yi Hwang (1501-1570). The number of movements signifies his birthplace on the 37th parallel of latitude.
Hwa-Rang	The military background of taekwondo stems from the Hwarang, the elite Sillian warriors of the 7th century. Going forward in time, its 29 movements pay homage to the Korean Army's 29th Infantry Division under General Choi.
Choong-Moo	Choong-Moo was the name given to one of the world's greatest naval tacticians, Admiral Sun Shin Yi (1545-1598). Built in 1592, his kobukson, or turtle boat, was the first iron-clad vessel built of its kind.
Kwang-Gae	The 39 movements of this *tul* represent the first two numerals in the year 391 AD when Kwang-Gae Toh Wang, who reclaimed the lost territories including much of Manchuria, gained the throne.

International Taekwon-Do Federation Tul Philosophy

(continued)

Tul	Philosophy
Po-Eun	This *tul* memorializes Chong Mong Chu whose pseudonym was Po-Eun. A loyal subject to the king, he also retains a place in Korean history as a famous poet and a pioneer in physics.
Ge-Baek	Securing his place in Korean, taekwondo and world history, this pattern immortalizes the famous Paekche general known by the same name for his severe and strict military discipline.
Eui-Am	Eui-Am, a pseudonym for Son Byong Hi, was a leader of the Korean independence movement of March 1, 1919. The movements within this *tul* represent his indomitable spirit in the service of his nation.
Choong-Jang	Kim Duk Ryang, also known as Choong-Jang, was a general during the Chosun Dynasty. This pattern symbolizes his death in prison at the young age of 27 before reaching full maturity.
Juche	A unique, Korean philosophy stating that man is the master of his own destiny, the pattern of Juche depicts that of Mount Baekdoo where deep within, it is said, this ideal is rooted.
Sam Il	Sam Il contains 33 movements representing the 33 patriots who planned the independence movement that began on March 1, 1919, targeted at unsettling the Japanese Occupation forces.
Yoo-Sin	The namesake of a commanding general during the Silla Dynasty, the 68 movements of this *tul* refer to last two numerals in the year 668 AD, the year Korea was finally unified.
Choi-Yong	General Choi Yong was Premier and Commander-in-Chief of the Koguryo armed forces during the 14th century, and was greatly respected for his humility, loyalty and patriotism.
Yon-Gae	Named after Koguryo General Yon Gae Somoon, the 49 motions that comprise this pattern symbolize the last two numerals in the year 649 AD. Destroying nearly 300,000 troops, the General evicted the Tang forces from Korea.
Ul-Ji	General Ul-Ji Moon Duk successfully defended the Korean nation against a Tang invasion force estimated at one million warriors. The 42 movements in this form represent General Choi, Hong Hi's age at the time of the *tul's* creation.

International Taekwon-Do Federation Tul Philosophy
(*continued*)

Tul	Philosophy
Moon-Moo	This pattern pays homage to Moon-Moo, the 30th king of the Silla Dynasty. According to his wishes, his body was remitted to the sea following his death "Where my soul shall forever defend my land against the Japanese."
So-San	This form commemorates the great monk Choi Hyong Ung (1520-1604) who in 1592 ad, organized a corps of warrior monks to repulse Japanese pirates who overran a majority of the Korean peninsula.
Se-Jong	Memorializing the most influential king in Korean history, the diagram of this pattern denotes king. Se-Jong is composed of 24 movements representing the 24 letters in hangul, the Korea alphabet, created by King Sejong in 1443.
Tong-Il	This, the last *tul* in the ITF series, represents the hope of unification by the people of the two Koreas which has been divided North and South since the end of World War II. The pattern of this form denotes one homogenous race.

example, the second *tul* in the series of twenty-four memorializes Tan-gun (c.2333 BC), the mythical progenitor of Korea, while the last, *Tong Il*, represents the future unification of the nation that was divided, north and south, in 1945 and sadly remains so today.

Some claim that superimposing a philosophical component over the physical practice of *poom-se* is at best a stretch of the imagination. However, this marriage presents a treasure trove for those seeking more than an aerobic workout from our training. Simply because taekwondo, with roots dating back to antiquity, was officially established in the 1950s, does not mean it cannot share in the ancient philosophical paradigms embraced by Asian culture as a whole. Korean society was greatly influenced by Buddhist and Confucian thought during the reign of the Silla, Koryo, and Chosun dynasties. So, why then should its native martial art not respectfully reflect this legacy in some way? Granted, Taoism played the least significant role in molding the nation's character. Yet even the South Korean flag, with the *Um/Yang* and its four trigrams, bears witness to the important contribution the *I Ching* and thus Taoism has had on the collective consciousness of the Korean people.

Today, some schools, especially those that feature mixed, non-traditional martial arts, have chosen to ignore the importance of the classic, formal exercises coupled with their philosophical foundation. If practiced at all, they are often relegated to a position

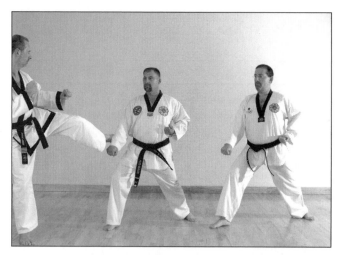

Figure 6-1

equal to that of warm-ups. Sadly, even the late Bruce Lee was heard to say that *poom-se* training is tantamount to "swimming on dry land." Still, metaphorically speaking, a contemporary painter applies brushstrokes from a palette of colors that have existed from time immemorial to create a canvas washed in art. What then is to preclude a modern martial artist from using ancient philosophical symbols to embellish his art?

Aside from the four phases of *poom-se* training examined above, the individual components contained within a form can be divided into three further categories, these being techniques that are obvious in intent, implied, or sometimes hidden within the sequences that comprise the *poom-se*.

A good example of an obvious technique is the hard, low block (*alle makki*) executed in the front stance (*ap koobi*) that launches the basic form, *Kicho Ilbo* (Figure 6-1). Another would be the double knife hand block (*dool sonnal momtang makki*) initiated at the beginning of *Taegeuk Sa Jang* (Figure 6-2). While I am certain a highly trained eye could prescribe addition defensive meaning to these motions, both techniques have a clear, singular intent; to intercept an incoming strike or kick aimed at the lower or middle portion of the body.

An implied technique would be one not depicted in training manuals, yet implicitly understood to occur in the mind of a competent practitioner during practical self-defense. A case in point could be a wrist grab that would follow the single knife hand block prior to a strike (*ahn han sonnal makki*) in the *poom-se Taegeuk Sam Jang* (Figure 6-3). In another scenario, a shoulder grab could potentially be executed once the double spread block (*doobal hecho makki*) in the form *Palgwe Yook Jang* is effective ly completed (Figure 6-4).

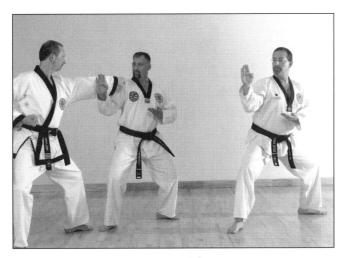

Figure 6-2

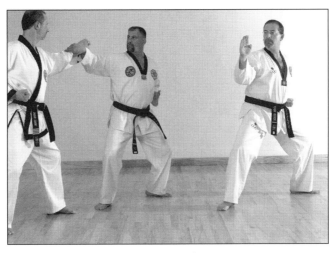

Figure 6-3

Furthermore, there exists a common belief that hidden techniques are buried within certain forms. The Japanese call these *okuden*. The source of this concept originated in times past when defensive skills within a form were, by necessity, intended to remain hidden from the eyes of invading armies, feuding clans, or vicious slave masters. As we have seen, the population of nations occupied by imperialistic forces were routinely forbidden to possess weapons of any kind and forced to rely on empty-hand martial arts skills to survive the brutal treatment meted out by their oppressors. Often, in order to preserve the potency of these defensive skills, practitioners would frequently disguise them as the movements of

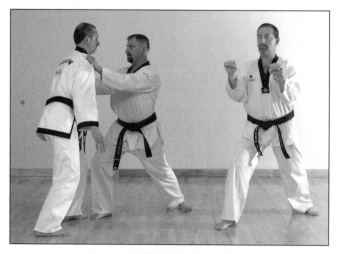

Figure 6-4

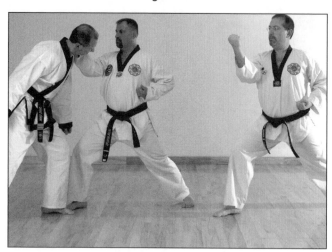

Figure 6-5

a dance. This is particularly true with the Brazilian martial art of *capoeira* where practitioners whirl and spin like dervishes while executing a unique collection of defensive kicks and strikes. Deceptively beautiful to watch, examples such as these remind us of the important role martial arts have played in the defense of suppressed citizens of downtrodden nations. An illustration of a hidden technique in modern day *poom-se* can be discerned in the form *Taegeuk Sa Jang* where the last middle block (*ahn momtang makki*) may also be a hammer fist (*me chumok*) to the head or ribs of the attacker (Figure 6-5).

Essential Elements of Poom-Se Training

- If possible, meditate on the philosophy and structure of the form prior to its execution.
- Memorize all discreet techniques and sequences within the form.
- In assuming the ready stance, express courage and confidence.
- When first learning the form, practice slowly and perform each technique with purpose.
- Look in the direction of the required movements.
- Be certain to give each stance the proper value it deserves.
- Visualize your target and execute each technique as if in an actual combat situation.
- Once you are familiar with the singular elements that comprise the form, practice to sequence.
- Relax and breathe with each movement while adding penetrating power to the end of each technique.
- Demonstrate both the soft and hard elements of the form, um and yang.
- Kihop vigorously, exhibiting a strong spirit when necessary.
- Once the individual movements and sequences of the form have been mastered, dwell on the philosophical component of the form during practice.
- Return to the ready stance with calm and grace once the form is completed.
- Practice the form in different surroundings so as not to be confused by a change in orientation.
- Practice only the forms that have been taught to you by a master instructor.

Years ago, prior to the worldwide proliferation of the martial arts through television and the cinema coupled with the opening of Eastern culture through international diplomacy, Asian masters chose to teach their students fewer forms but in greater detail, going deep rather than wide so to speak. In fact, it is said that a form cannot be truly internalized until it has been performed hundreds if not thousands of times. Clearly, this is not the case today with most fourth-dan master instructors required to commit to memory as many as thirty to forty *poom-se*. Furthermore, it is said that masters of the past would transmit forms to their students in layers with the most trusted pupils receiving the full potential of each technique once they have demonstrated their dedication to the art. Either way, it is clear that forms have played a major role in the transmission of martial arts skills for centuries. To ignore or discount this component of the traditional taekwondo curriculum, along with the underlying philosophy mirrored in *poom-se*, would be a great disservice not only to students presently training, but also to those still to come. Regardless of the mode by which a *poom-se* is captured for posterity, whether it is of a physical or electronic nature, it is ultimately the responsibility of today's instructors to cherish, preserve, and transmit the classic forms uncorrupted by lack of knowledge or personal style. Only then are practitioners of the future certain to benefit from this effective and traditional form of self-defense education.

PART THREE

Technique

CHAPTER 7
Physical Conditioning for Martial Arts

Prior to beginning any intense physical activity, particularly martial arts, it is wise to prepare the body both externally and internally for the challenges that lay ahead. External exercises condition the striking and blocking surfaces of the body including the hands, forearms, legs and feet. Conversely, internal preparation entails warming the body's core through aerobic activity while enriching the muscles, tendons, and ligaments with a fresh supply of blood to reduce the likelihood of injury. Once this is accomplished, the practitioner can then safely advance to exercises that promote strength and flexibility, a much-needed element for meaningful taekwondo practice.

Whereas internal preparation is a constant prelude to every training session, external conditioning requires progressive practice over long periods of time in order to prove effective. One cannot expect to receive a blow of any magnitude with equanimity, or break a solid object with the hands or feet in an effort to develop focus and indomitable will, without first performing a regimen of exercises aimed at conditioning strategic areas of the body. Often various types of training equipment are employed to accomplish this goal. One such device is the *makiwara* (Figure 7-1). Originally a straw-padded striking post, the *makiwara* found in most *dojangs* today consists of a piece of canvas-covered foam mounted on a strip of wood. It is primarily used to develop the fists and edges of the hand. Assuming an appropriate stance, the practitioner strikes the *makiwara* repeatedly, conditioning the intended point of the body in the process. Any number of techniques can be practiced in this manner

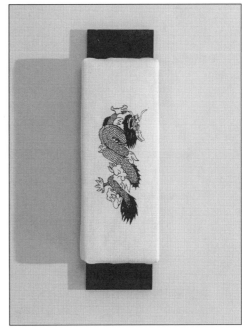

Figure 7-1

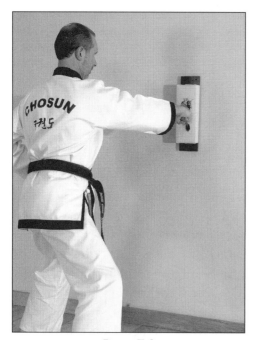

Figure 7-2

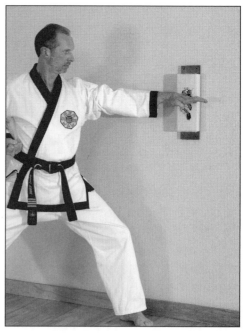

Figure 7-3

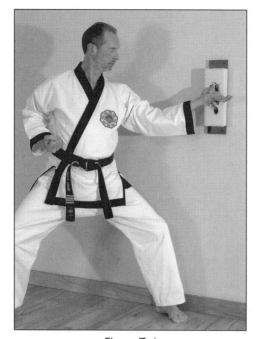

Figure 7-4

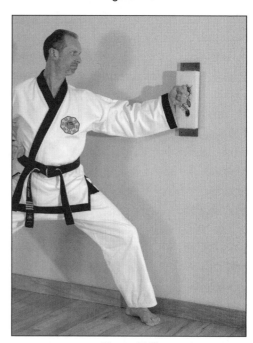

Figure 7-5

including the fore fist (Figure 7-2), knife hand (Figure 7-3), ridge hand (Figure 7-4), and back fist (Figure 7-5).

CONDITIONING DRILLS

In an effort to improve kicking techniques, in addition to conditioning the striking surface of the foot, heavy bags, focus pads, and kicking shields are frequently used. The kicking shield is a useful tool in developing a strong side kick (Figure 7-6), round kick (Figure 7-7), or back kick (Figure 7-8). Focus pads are relied upon when the martial artist chooses to concentrate on striking at a

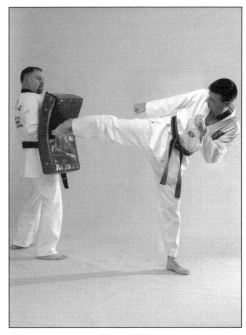

Figure 7-6

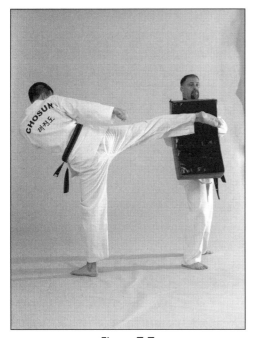

Figure 7-7

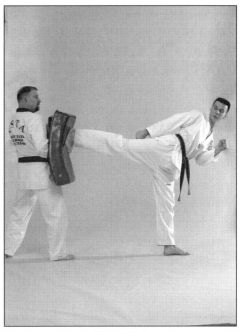

Figure 7-8

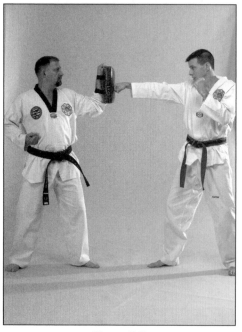

Figure 7-9

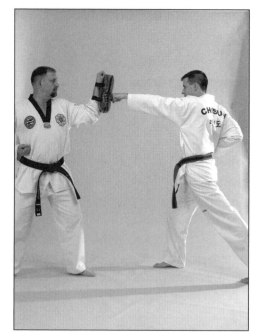

Figure 7-10

single point in space. Training mitts held by a partner will prove effective in practicing any of the aforementioned hand techniques as well as the jab/reverse punch combination (Figures 7-9 and 7-10). Similarly, kicking paddles provide a target for many of the kicks mentioned above as well as jumping and spinning kicks (Figures 7-11 and 7-12).

Conditioning the forearm to accept a sudden strike is a more difficult task and, therefore, requires some imagination when creating drills that harden this portion of the body. A partner drill that has proven effective in not only conditioning the forearm, but in enhancing focus and stamina, has two students facing one another. Student A assumes an appropriate stance in conjunction with a desired blocking technique. Student B then steps into the same stance and executes the same block only mirror image (Figure 7-13). Student A then steps forward initiating the block as student B steps back doing the same (Figure 7-14). This motion is continued for the length of the training hall. Once the students reach the opposite end of the room, their roles are reversed with student B stepping forward while A steps back. This drill can be repeated with any number of forearm blocking techniques. An inside to outside middle block (*bakat momtong makki*) in back stance (*dwi koobi*) is illustrated here for demonstration purposes. If training space is at a premium, static drills exist

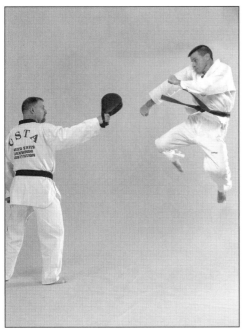

Figure 7-11

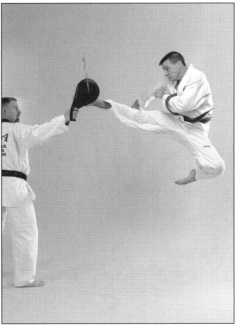

Figure 7-12

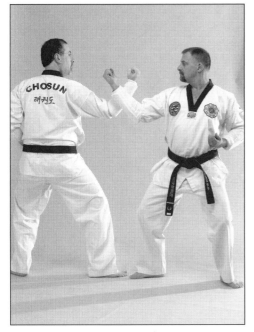

Figure 7-13

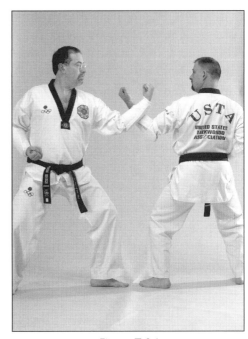

Figure 7-14

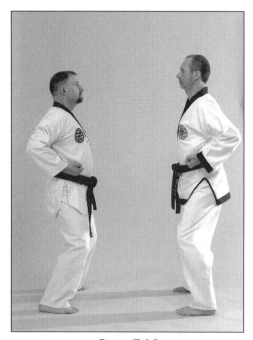

Figure 7-15

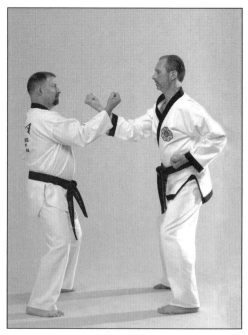

Figure 7-16

that serve a similar purpose. In this exercise, student A and student B face each other seated in a horse stance (*ja choom sogi*) (Figure 7-15). Using the right forearm first, both students execute an outside-to-inside middle block (*ahn momtong makki*) (Figure 7-16). Once contact is made, the right arm completes a downward arc ending in a low block (Figure 7-17). At this point, both students switch to the left arm repeating the blocking techniques (Figures 7-18 and 7-19). The exercise is then continued, alternating between the right and left arms.

The intensity with which blocks and strikes are delivered during practice is a function of self-control, respect, and cooperation between partners. It is important

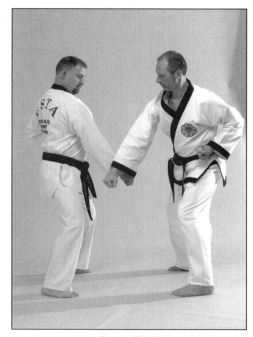

Figure 7-17

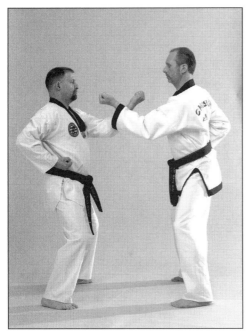

Figure 7-18

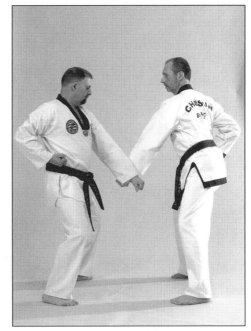

Figure 7-19

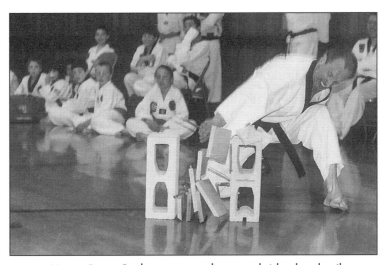

Master Doug Cook executes a downward ridge hand strike
through multiple pieces of wood during a USTA demonstration.

to note that a danger exists of interrupting the flow of *Ki* traveling through complimentary meridians in the arms. Care should be taken to massage the forearms following the completion of each drill to restore this flow. To avoid bruising or excessive

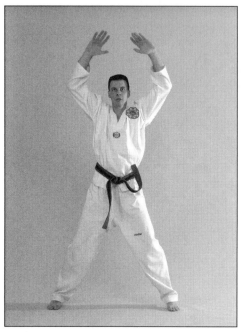

Figure 7-20

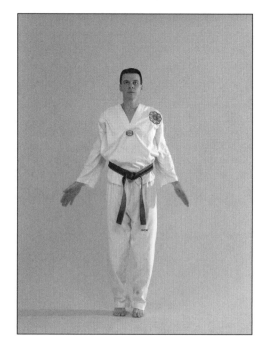

Figure 7-21

stress to the arms, it is recommended that fabric forearm guards be worn by both participants.

External conditioning requires determination and patience on the part of the taekwondoist since the net results are neither quickly apparent nor necessarily comfortable. Conditioning the anatomy is a long-time endeavor that must be approached slowly in order to develop strong striking and blocking surfaces. The practitioner should always be aware of the dangers from calcification resulting from repeated strikes that can eventually lead to arthritis or nerve damage.

External and internal conditioning exercises are not exclusive of one another, but must be practiced and sustained in tandem. If external conditioning hopes of prevent the startle-flinch reaction to an unprovoked attack by preparing the martial artist to manage the impact of a strike, then it can be said that aerobic, flexibility, and strengthening drills maximize the body for a quick and effective counterattack.

Using the analogy of a sponge, which is far easier to tear when it is dry rather than moist, we can appreciate the importance of aerobic exercises that increase circulation to the body's connective tissue. The most common exercise used to enhance cardiovascular performance and encourage blood flow in the athlete prior to flexibility training tends to be jumping jacks (Figures 7-20 and 7-21). Other exercises that

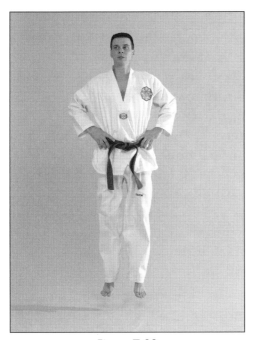

Figure 7-22

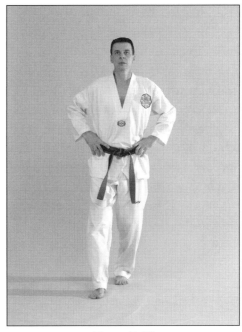

Figure 7-23

serve the same purpose might be jogging around the perimeter of the *dojang* or executing a series of bounces, forward-steps, and cross-steps in place (Figures 7-22, 7-23, and 7-24). Additionally, some students may choose to jump rope before class commences. Naturally, before any vigorous exercise is attempted, the student should inform the instructor of any preexisting medical condition that may cause a problem or result in a health emergency.

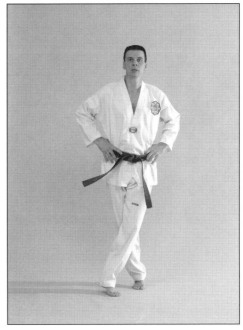

Figure 7-24

FLEXIBILITY DRILLS

Once the muscles have been aerobically fed, flexibility drills can follow. These exercises should be recognized as an essential component of any class since martial arts techniques have the potential of imposing extreme stress on the joints of the body. A sufficient period of time, anywhere from 10 to 20 minutes, should be allocated in an effort to prevent injury by stretching the entire body.

Flexibility drills vary greatly from instructor to instructor and from school to school. The series of exercises, depicted here in their recommended order of performance, are commonly practiced and if done correctly will promote a safe training experience. Each movement should be held or repeated for a count of ten.

Neck: Inhale and bring the right ear to the right shoulder. Exhale and tilt the chin to the chest. Inhale and bring the left ear to the left shoulder. Exhale and tilt the head to the rear. (Figures 7-25, 7-26, 7-27, and 7-28).

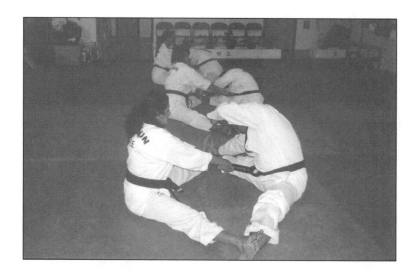

Students perform flexibility exercises prior to training.

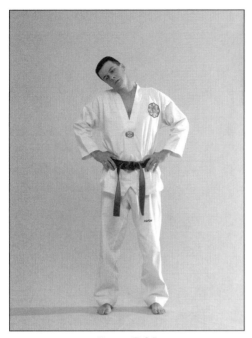

Figure 7-25

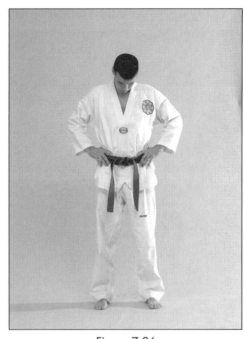

Figure 7-26

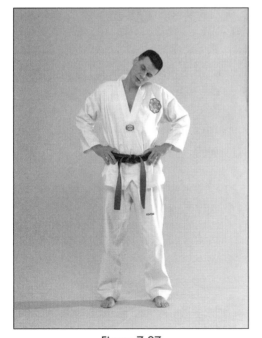

Figure 7-27

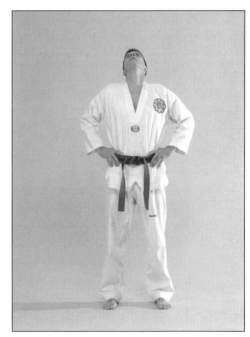

Figure 7-28

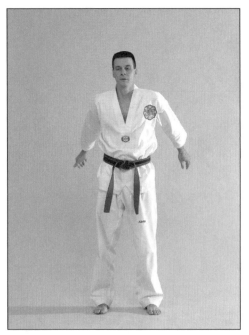

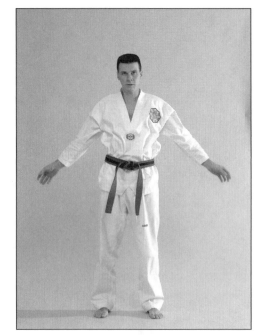

Figure 7-29   Figure 7-30

Arms: Swing both arms simultaneously backwards and forwards in a circular motion towards the front and rear of the body. (Figures 7-29 and 7-30)

Side Stretch: With feet shoulder width apart and right hand on the right hip, extend the left arm straight up, palm open. Allowing the elbow to bend slightly, tilt and stretch the upper torso to the right side. Repeat using the right arm. (Figures 7-31 and 7-32)

Hips: With both hands on the hips, feet shoulder width apart, rotate the hips first clockwise, and then counterclockwise. The head and feet remain stationary. (Figure 7-33)

Knees: With feet together, bend and place the hands on the knees. Rotate the knees first clockwise, and then counterclockwise. (Figure 7-34)

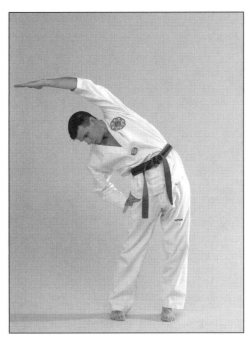

Figure 7-31

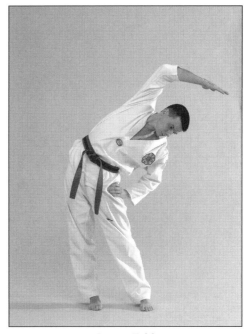

Figure 7-32

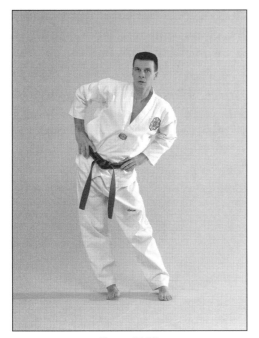

Figure 7-33

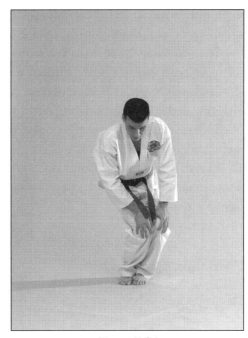

Figure 7-34

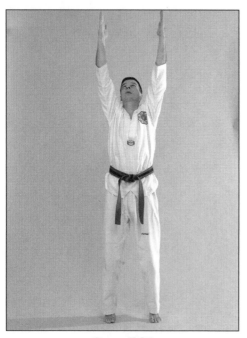

Figure 7-35

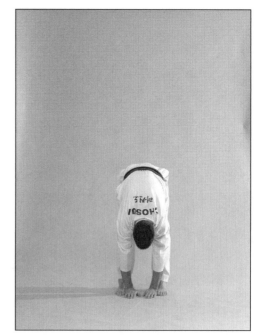

Figure 7-36

Upper Stretch: With both arms extended straight over the head, feet shoulder width apart, reach up coming off the heels with each movement. (Figure 7-35)

Back Stretch: Bend forward from the waist, locking the knees and pressing the palms to the floor. (Figure 7-36)

Stomach Stretch: With the hands on the hips, bend backwards tucking the chin into the chest. (Figure 7-37)

Twists: Assuming a horse stance, lift both elbows to shoulder height, fists facing each other. Twist twice to the right and twice to the left. (Figures 7-38 and 7-39)

Hamstring Stretch: Bend the right knee while keeping the right foot flat on the floor. Extend the left leg out to the side toes facing upward. Repeat on the opposite side.

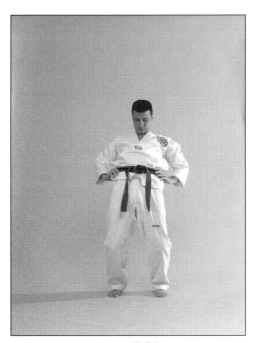

Figure 7-37

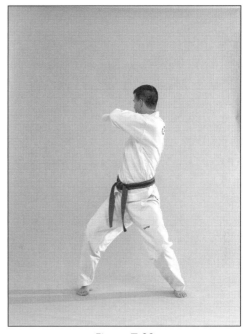

Figure 7-38

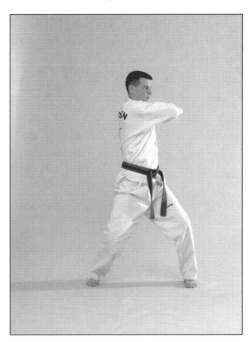

Figure 7-39

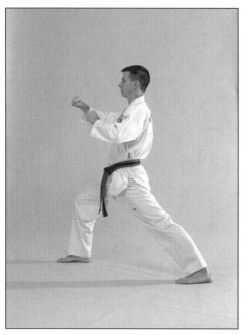

Figure 7-40

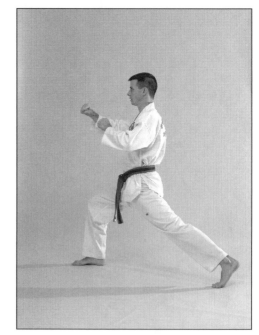

Figure 7-41

Front Stance Stretch: a. Step into a front stance with the right leg. Bring the hands up in a fighting position. b. Remain in the same position but lift the heel of the left foot. c. Placing the left hand on the floor for support, bring the right hand in and around the back of the right foot placing it palm down on the outside. Repeat in the opposite direction. (Figures 7-40, 7-41, and 7-42)

Straddle Stretch: a. Open the legs double shoulder width apart. With both hands, reach down and across to the right ankle bringing the forehead down to the right knee. b. Repeat on the left side. c. Bringing the head down to the center, place the right hand on the right ankle and the left hand on the left ankle. (Figures 7-43, 7-44, and 7-45)

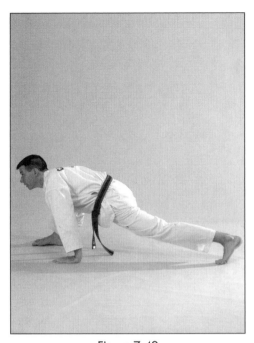

Figure 7-42

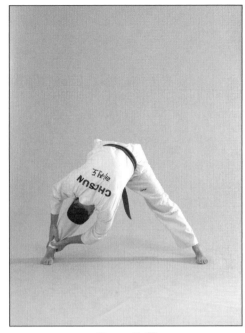

Figure 7-43

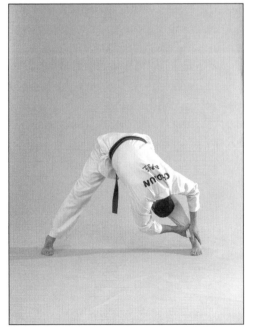

Figure 7-44

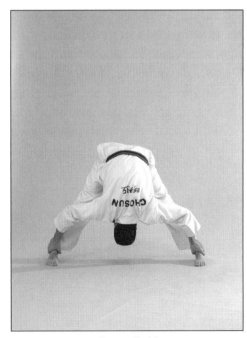

Figure 7-45

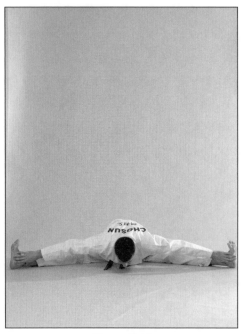

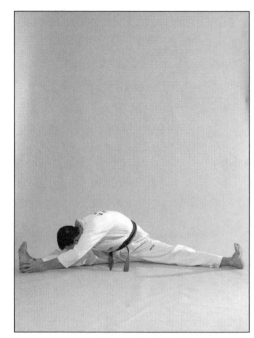

Figure 7-46   Figure 7-47

Seated Split Stretch: a. Seated on the floor, open the legs as wide as possible, toes facing upward. Bend from the small of the back while reaching for the right foot with the right hand and the left foot with the left hand. b. Turn the torso to the right and reach both hands to the right foot. c. Repeat on the opposite side. (7-46, 7-47, and 7-48)

Butterfly Stretch: a. Sitting erect, bring the soles of the feet together with the heels as close to the groin as possible. Slowly flex the knees upward and downward. b. Bending from the waist, bring the forehead down to the feet. (Figures 7-49 and 7-50)

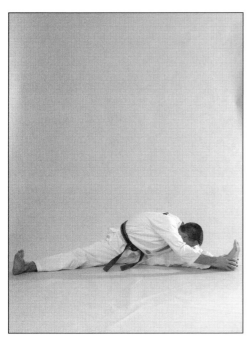

Figure 7-48

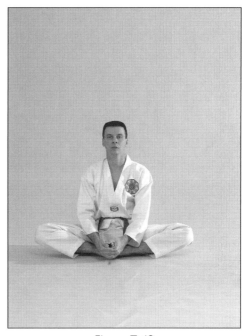

Figure 7-49

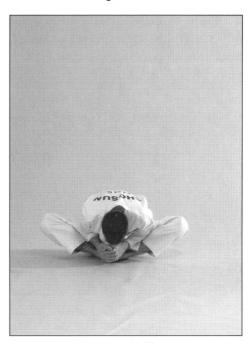

Figure 7-50

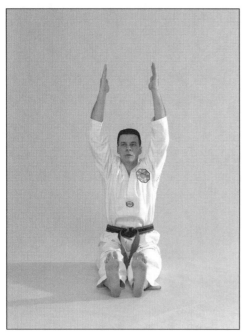

Figure 7-51

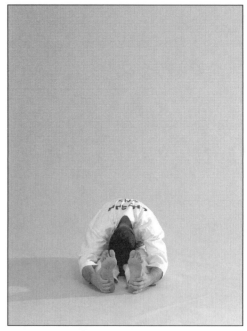

Figure 7-52

Front Stretch: a. Sitting erect, extend the legs straight out from the body, feet together and toes facing upward, and then lift the arms above the head palms facing each other. b. Slowly bend forward from the waist reaching for the toes or ankles. (Figures 7-51 and 7-52)

Leg & Ankle Stretch: a. With both legs extended from the body and the back straight, take the left ankle and place it on the right knee. b. Rotate the left foot with the right hand, clockwise and the counterclockwise. c. Rotate the toes. d. Take hold of the left heel with the left hand and lock it straight out. e. Retract the left leg and stretch it out to the left side. Repeat the exercise by placing the right ankle on the left knee. (Figures 7-53, 7-54, 7-55, 7-56, and 7-57)

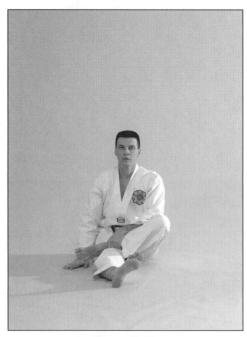

Figure 7-53

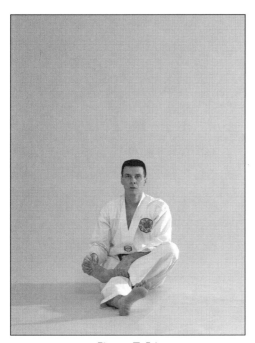

Figure 7-54

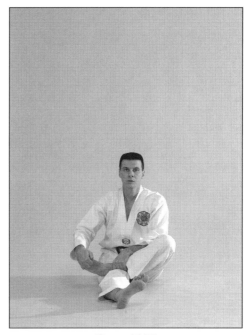

Figure 7-55

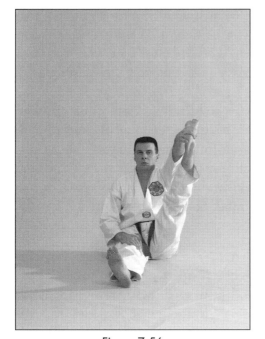

Figure 7-56

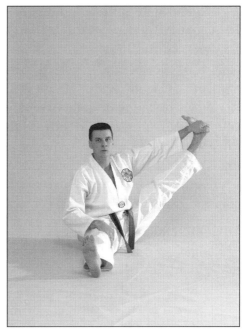

Figure 7-57

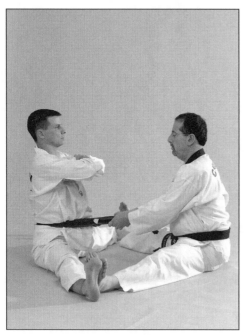

Figure 7-58

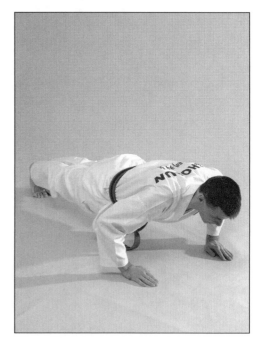

Figure 7-59

Partner Split Stretch: Student A sits across from student B with legs open, toes facing upward and arms crossed in front of the chest. Student B gently pushes A's legs outward with his heels while pulling on his belt. The stretch is held for a count of ten, then released and repeated. Student A then performs the same exercise on Student B. (Figure 7-58)

When executing flexibility exercises, remember to breathe naturally and not hold your breath. Moreover, surrender to the stretch, visualizing the muscles elongating in the process. Be aware of your limits; as *taiji* master Jou Tsung Hwa was fond of saying, "strive to make a little progress" at each training session rather than by putting your body in jeopardy from overstretching. Taekwondo training is progressive to the core and, with diligent practice, a strong and limber body will be realized.

STRENGTHENING EXERCISES

Time permitting, a short period of strengthening exercises often follow flexibility drills during a training session. While free-weight lifting focuses on muscle development and sculpting, it is time consuming and, if desired, best practiced separate from martial arts class. In place of this however, performing a short series of push-ups, crunches, and leg raises can satisfactorily complete the required regimen of conditioning exercises prior to taekwondo training.

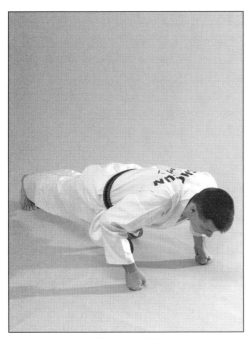

Figure 7-60

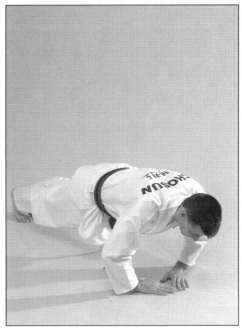

Figure 7-61

Push ups can be executed while supporting oneself on the palms (Figure 7-59), knuckles (Figure 7-60), or by creating a diamond pattern with the thumbs and index fingers touching (Figure 7-61). If a training partner is available, the student may have them hold their legs at the ankles similar to the way a wheelbarrow would be lifted. Push-ups are then practiced from this angle (Figure 7-62). Care should be taken not to release the legs too suddenly which may result in injury.

Crunches, or sit-ups, can also be done solo or with a partner. If carried out with a partner, student A can lock their insteps behind the calves of student B, with student

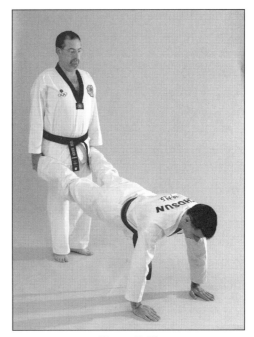

Figure 7-62

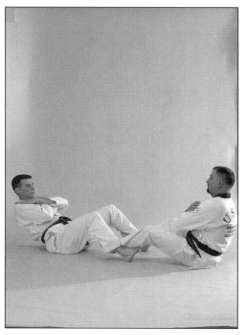

Figure 7-63

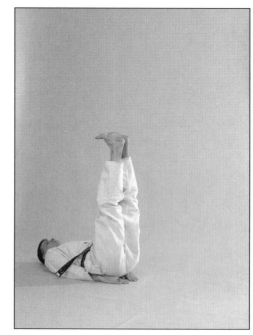

Figure 7-64

B doing likewise (Figure 7-63). Sit-ups should be done slowly, in shallow throws, thus preventing the torso from resting as would be the case if the chest were to be incorrectly raised fully upright, or lowered to make contact with the floor. Performing sit-ups in this manner is not only safer and surprisingly easier, but also more physically rewarding.

Leg raises, or lifts, are used to strengthen the muscles in the abdomen. Lying on the floor with the hands placed under the buttocks to support the back, the student repeatedly raises and lowers the legs from a few inches off the ground to a ninety-degree position relative to the floor (Figure 7-64). It is important to keep the knees locked out, while not allowing the heels to touch the ground as the legs come downward. After approximately ten leg lifts, a scissor pattern can be executed (Figure 7-65), followed by a series of circles, clockwise and then counterclockwise (Figure 7-66). A modification of this exercise involves the use of a partner who straddles student A's head while A is lying on the floor. Student A then holds student B's ankles while B pushes A's legs forward (Figure 7-67). As soon as the legs are a few inches off the floor, student A quickly raises them to the ninety-degree position (Figure 7-68). Repeat the cycle anywhere from ten to twenty times.

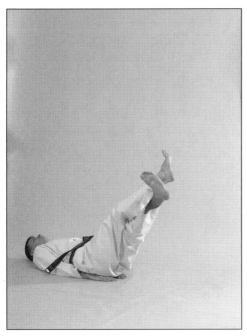

Figure 7-65

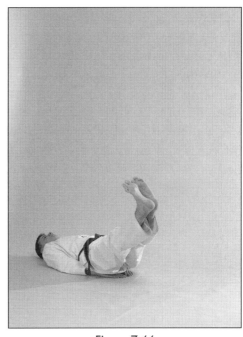

Figure 7-66

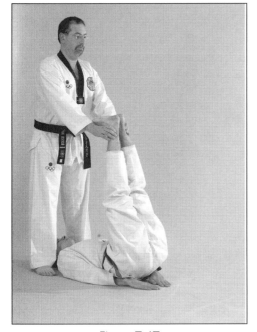

Figure 7-67

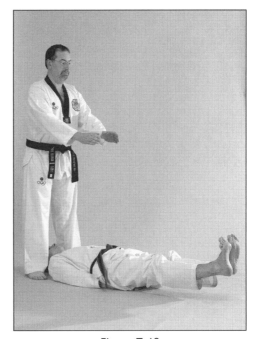

Figure 7-68

SUMMARY

Physical conditioning exercises act as an overture for intense martial arts training. They stretch and strengthen the body for the kicking, striking, and blocking techniques that are the hallmark of traditional taekwondo. Without these drills, the martial artist is in peril of suffering torn ligaments, cramped muscles, and weakened blocking surfaces. Clearly, it is not enough simply to become proficient in the defensive and offensive movements of taekwondo; one must also develop physically, both internally and externally, for the rigors diligent martial arts training demands of the body.

CHAPTER 8

Training Methods in Traditional Taekwondo

Clearly, if practiced in a traditional manner, taekwondo has proven to be an extremely effective means of self-defense. However, skills of this sort are not developed overnight. For the most part, years of diligent training are required to condition the body, fortify the spirit, and enrich the mind in preparation for precise, focused technique. How, then, does the sincere practitioner reach this point of proficiency?

Realistic self-defense training in anticipation of an unprovoked attack is difficult at best. One cannot accurately predict the terrain, time of day, or weapon of choice whether it be knife, firearm, or something as common as a trash can lid, unique to a given altercation. Compound this with the fact that one's temperament is rarely consistent from day to day, and the true nature of this dilemma begins to emerge. Still, in the eyes of the martial artist, it is better to be prepared through a regimen of conscientious practice, than to fall victim to the misdirected vengeance of a bellicose aggressor. Yet, if one were to respond to a mock attack in the training environment with maximum effort and power, it is likely that one's daily routine would often be interrupted due to serious injury. With this in mind, the founders of taekwondo provided several ritualistic methods of drilling between pairs of students that allows one participant to assume the role of the aggressor while the other counters with an appropriate defense and counterattack. Not only do these scenarios address the physical requirements of self-defense practice, but bundle in the philosophical considerations as well.

The first component of the taekwondo defensive syllabus that we shall examine is traditionally referred to as *il su sik*, or one-step sparring. A modern label for the same body of techniques, adopted by practitioners of WTF-style taekwondo, is *han bon kyorugi*. Since my training is rooted in traditional taekwondo, I will use the former phrase throughout this work. One-step sparring strategy, at least for the most part, prepares the student to defend against the lunge punch, perhaps the most prevalent offensive tool common to nearly all confrontations. This by no means excludes defense against other related instruments of attack such as the front kick or round kick. In addition to one-step sparring, the student often practices *sam su sik* or three-step sparring, with similar results.

Likewise, another segment of the traditional core curriculum that we will study focuses on *ho sin sool* or self-defense techniques. While *il su sik* provides solutions against strikes, *ho sin sool,* conversely, is concerned with defending against various grabs including, but not exclusive to, headlocks, bear hugs, the full nelson, cross hand grabs, shoulder grabs, and same side grabs. Weapon defense, too, plays an important role in *ho sin sool* practice.

Although this volume focuses mainly on *il su sik* and *ho sin sool* techniques, still another facet that nurtures the defensive capabilities of the taekwondoist is that of *prearranged* and *free sparring*. It should be pointed out that in years past, the bulk of martial arts training was handed down through the practice of the classical forms or *poom-se* as described earlier. Sport sparring was rare or virtually non-existent; if the martial artist fought at all it was for self-preservation. Free sparring today, however, coupled with the use of innovative safety equipment, teaches the student how to turn a threatening situation to his advantage through the use of superior strategy and a strong will. Naturally, in today's sport-oriented society, it is often used as a means of competition and entertainment.

Were it not for the ritualized practice of *il su sik*, *ho sin sool*, prearranged, and free sparring, self-defense practice holds the potential of being a chaotic and painful pursuit. Most martial artists due to the very nature of their art learn to accept a modicum of discomfort in the course of their training. This discomfort does not mean that they take pleasure from it nor does it exempt them from injury. As we shall see in greater detail, the sincere practitioner of traditional taekwondo by using the above training strategies will develop an understanding of safety, courtesy, knowledge of distancing, power, body mechanics, breath control, use of *Ki,* presence of mind, and a deep appreciation for the true essence of martial arts doctrine.

IL SU SIK: ONE-STEP SPARRING

The diligent performance of *il su sik* serves a variety of purposes. Primarily, it permits the student of taekwondo to practice predetermined defensive tactics against an opponent confident that there is little danger of injury. This last point assumes both parties are adroit in the basic technique of striking, blocking, sweeping, and falling correctly. Subsequently, since there is seldom any hard contact made, practitioners of all ages and gender can benefit from this type of training. The term "one-step sparring" is derived from the fact that the aggressor advances one step forward while

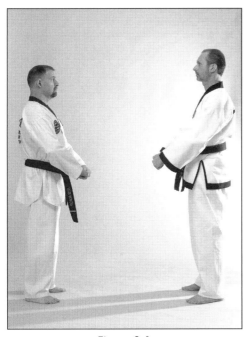

Figure 8-1

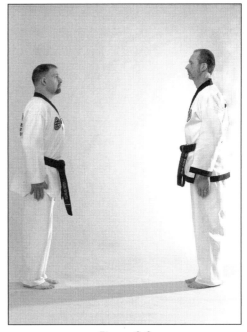

Figure 8-2

attacking prior to the defender initiating an appropriate defense. The drill consists of two students facing one another at a minimum distance of three feet, with a maximum distance not to exceed the height of the tallest participant. The students are then instructed to assume the ready stance (*joombi*) (Figure 8-1), followed by attention stance (*cha riot*) (Figure 8-2), and then, bow (*kyungye*) (Figure 8-3).

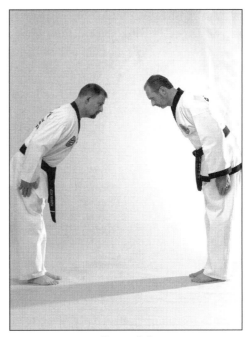

Figure 8-3

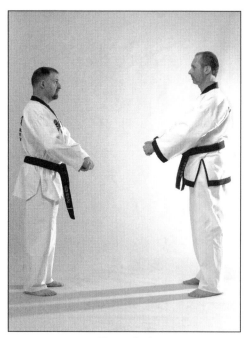

Figure 8-4

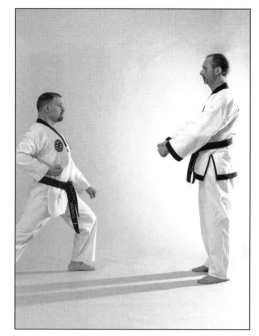

Figure 8-5

At this point, both will return to the ready stance (Figure 8-4), and the instructor will introduce the drill by announcing *"il su sik!"* The students will respond to this command by replying *"il su sik, Sir!"* After confirming proper distancing, one of the pair, being assigned the task of attacker, will step back with the right leg into a front stance (*ap koobi*) and signify his intent to strike by shouting *"kihop"* while simultaneously executing a left low block (*ahre makki*) (Figure 8-5). The defender will then yell *"kihop"* in return signaling his preparedness to defend. The aggressor, advancing one step forward, shouts *"kihop"* once again, and executes a predetermined strike, in this case a middle punch (*momtang juluki*) (Figure 8-6). Consequently, the defending student will mount a combination defensive/offensive technique commensurate with their level of proficiency (Figure 8-7).

One-step sparring can be thought of as bridging the gap between the dynamic self-defense practice offered by *poom-se* and the more realistic spontaneity of free sparring. Practiced slowly at first and with purpose, it is a proven method of overcoming the "startle-flinch" reaction. This is a response, founded in self-preservation, whereby the individual is overcome with surprise by an incoming attack and thus unable to defend effectively, a truly dangerous situation for the experienced martial artist. Furthermore, the ritualistic self-defense drill of *il su sik*, while artificial in

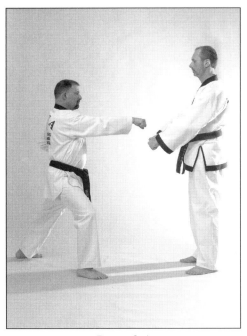

Figure 8-6

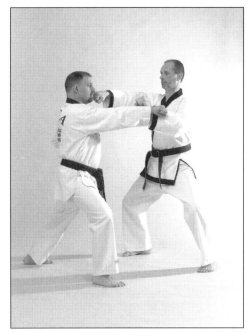

Figure 8-7

nature, is steeped in tradition and safety. Not exclusive to taekwondo, the value of *il su sik* practice is evident since it is practiced throughout the martial arts community in the related disciplines of Korean, Okinawan, and Japanese descent.

SAM SU SIK: THREE-STEP SPARRING

The parameters that apply to il su sik practice relate equally to sam su sik or three-step sparring drills. Known in modern nomenclature a *sam bon kyorugi,* the main difference here is that rather than advancing a single step forward with a pre-arranged offensive technique, the attacker advances three steps forward with an offending strike. Three-step sparring provides the beginner with an additional few seconds to consider his counterattack. Likewise, the advanced martial artist can benefit from sam su sik practice by having the attacker initiate three different offending techniques. The initial four sam su sik techniques depicted in this book revolve around defense against the high lunge punch with the final four centering on defense against the middle lunge punch. After becoming familiar with the rhythm of sam su sik practice, the taekwondoist can begin to improvise defensive strategies against a variety of techniques.

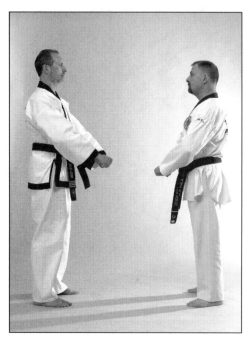

Figure 8-8

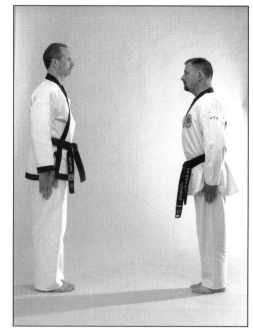

Figure 8-9

HO SIN SOOL: SELF-DEFENSE TECHNIQUES

Many of the *ho sin sool* techniques depicted in this book can be traced back to those found in hapkido, a martial art of Korean origin related to taekwondo, aikido a Japanese discipline founded by Morihei Ueshiba, and judo created by Jigoro Kano. These defensive strategies routinely rely on balance, knowledge of pressure points, and circular motions largely borrowed from the Chinese fighting arts. The martial artist employs these biomechanical principles when executing the throws, sweeps, and joint locks unique to this form of self-defense. In practicing *ho sin sool*, it is essential that the aggressor signal the extent of the defenders effectiveness by "tapping out." If this safeguard is not observed it is likely that injury will ensue. The ritual practice of *ho sin sool* is similar to that of *il su sik*. The students are again instructed to assume the ready stance (*joombi*) (Figure 8-8), followed by attention stance (*cha riot*) (Figure 8-9). Following the bow of courtesy (*kyungye*) (Figure 8-10) both will return to the ready stance (Figure 8-11). The instructor will then initiate the drill with the command, *"ho sin sool!"* The students will respond by replying *"ho sin sool, Sir!"* The assigned attacker will then assail his partner with a pre-arranged attack (Figure 8-12) quickly followed by the defender responding with an appropriate defense (Figure 8-13). Once the defensive technique is deemed effective, the

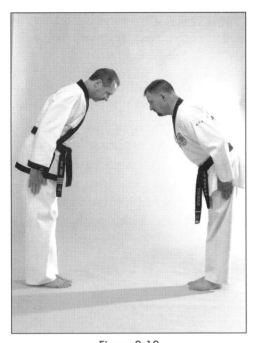

Figure 8-10

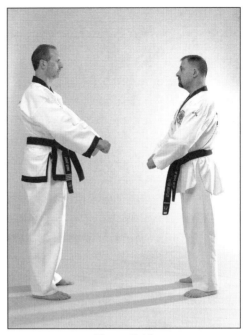

Figure 8-11

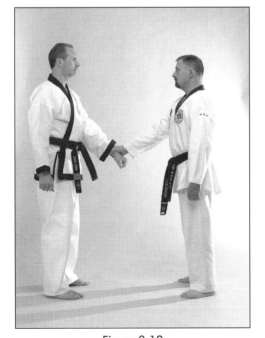

Figure 8-12

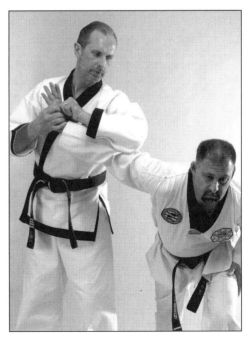

Figure 8-13

attacker will signal by tapping out. It is imperative that a great deal of courtesy is displayed between partners so that each may practice effectively and with safety.

PREARRANGED SPARRING

This component of the taekwondo curriculum is a link between static self-defense drills and situations of a more realistic nature. While still controlled, pre-arranged sparring permits the practitioner to move dynamically, altering both the stances and the order in which techniques are delivered in the process. As in *il su sik* and *ho sin sool*, pairs of students, usually clad in safety gear, are alternately assigned the role of attacker and defender. Since little or no contact is permitted, the practitioner can perform sequenced techniques of their choice that are appropriate for their body style. Prearranged sparring allows the taekwondoist to test his strengths safely while refining his weaknesses. (See Figures 8-14 through 8-21)

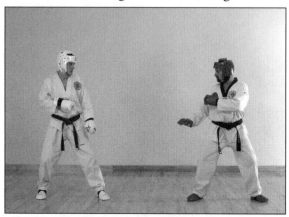

Figure 8-14

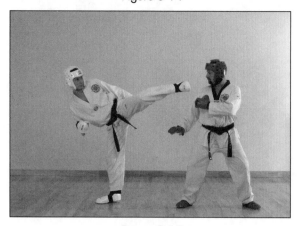

Figure 8-15

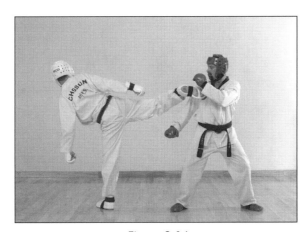

Figure 8-16

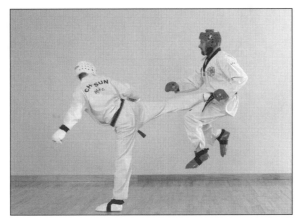

Figure 8-17

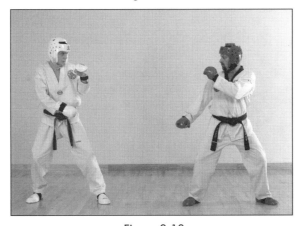

Figure 8-18

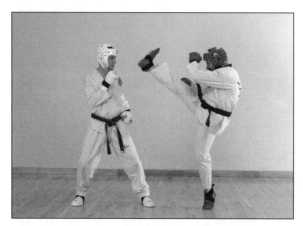

Figure 8-19

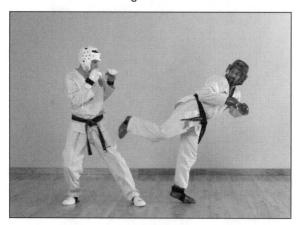

Figure 8-20

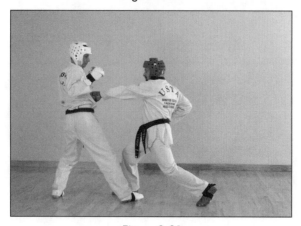

Figure 8-21

FREE SPARRING

For the most part, free sparring permits the student to utilize martial arts skills in an unrestrained fashion without regard for predetermined sequences unlike *il su sik*, *ho sin sool*, or prearranged sparring. In most cases, however, even this form of defensive training is limited in scope due to safety and regulatory issues. For instance, sweeps, kicks below the belt and hand strikes to the face, techniques clearly of defensive value, are largely discouraged since free sparring more than not is intended as a method of preparing the practitioner for sport competition. Techniques of the type mentioned above are not awarded points in games governed by World Taekwondo Federation rules and are therefore frequently eliminated from practice for this reason. Considering there exists approximately 3200 techniques in traditional taekwondo according to General Choi, Hong Hi, this approach clearly short circuits the defensive process. However, as mentioned earlier, sparring results in the practitioner learning how to cope with stressful situations by using strategy to effectively resolve these matters. Since this work is largely committed to the demonstration of self-defense tactics involving sweeps, throws, and strikes not necessarily sanctioned in the sports world, we will be focusing primarily on the practical application of *il su sik* and *ho sin sool* techniques rather than those of prearranged or free sparring. (See Figures 8-22 through 8-29)

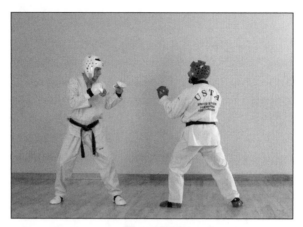

Figure 8-22

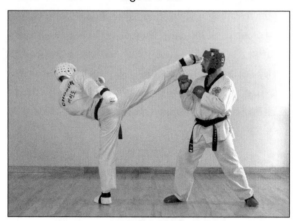

Figure 8-23

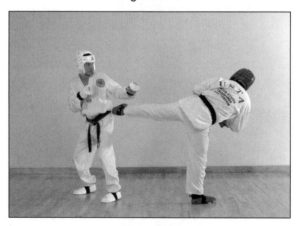

Figure 8-24

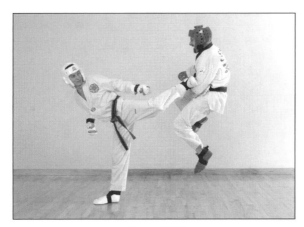

Figure 8-25

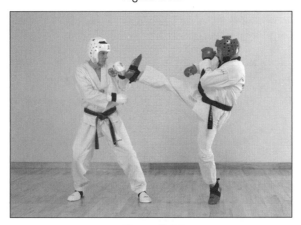

Figure 8-26

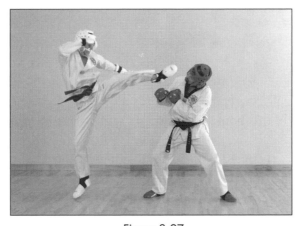

Figure 8-27

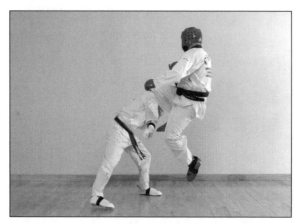

Figure 8-28

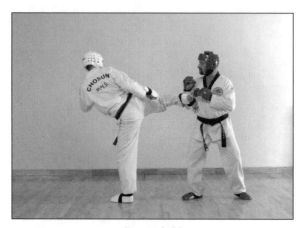

Figure 8-29

COLLATERAL BENEFITS OF PRACTICE

Aside from the obvious defensive value associated with the aforementioned training paradigms, over time supplementary aspects of significance will be reveled to the practitioner through diligent practice of *il su sik* and *ho sin sool*. Refining these peripheral qualities will greatly enhance one's ability to execute effectively the technique demonstrated in this book. Let us then examine the most prevalent of these in some detail.

Courtesy: At first, it may be difficult to equate the virtue of courtesy with the aggressive nature of martial arts training. However, without courtesy effective practice would almost be impossible. Starting with the initial bow at the beginning of class to the attitude expressed by the novice toward senior belts, this attribute plays a major role in the safety and ritual of taekwondo. Likewise, the courtesy articulated in the *dojang* is carried forth in daily life reinforcing the virtue of humility, yet another essential element of taekwondo.

Self-Control: If the purpose of diligent training is to improve the efficiency of self-defense preparedness, then it is essential that the practitioner devote himself to precise, practical technique. This said, strikes should be executed with sufficient power to terminate a confrontation with a single blow. In Korean, this principle is known as *il kyuk pil sul*, or "first strike, swift kill." Considering that relatively little pressure is required to break a bone and that technique should be practiced at reasonably close proximity to the objective in order to be effective, great care must be taken to avoid excessive contact. This minute zone of safety is governed by self-control and, as any student knows, demonstrates the difference between the novice and experienced practitioner.

Distancing: Clearly, a hand strike or kick will prove effective only if it comes in contact with its intended target. Therefore, the martial artist must adapt technique to fit the length of the arms and legs, which are the primary defensive tools. It follows that just as a great mountain tapers to a peak, so the kinetic energy of a strike or kick should terminate in an explosive apex of power coupled with penetrating force. Finding the precise distance one must be from the target is crucial to this principle. Over-reaching with a technique will result in a severe dissipation of power prior to impact. Likewise, being too close in proximity to the target will limit the trajectory of a strike precluding the complete development of power. Moreover, the practitioner needs to consider the proper footwork required to provide stability when stepping into appropriate stances. The stance is like the roots of a tree. If it is too shallow, the defender will stumble, and the technique will falter. Every limb of the body must cooperate to deliver maximum power and stability.

Ki **Development:** Knowledge of this topic plays a significant role in the holistic maturity of the martial artist as we have seen in a previous section of this book devoted to its coverage. However, it is important to remember that in Asian culture and traditional Chinese medicine in particular, it is believed that life is sustained by the internal life force know as *Ki* in Korean and Japanese, or *Chi* in Chinese. Manipulation of this vital energy by the martial artist can support technique many fold or, in the converse, offer relief from injury. Through concentrated effort, one can learn how to direct the flow of *Ki* to various parts of the body thus creating a shield against harm while projecting its potential energy through the fist or foot to intensify a strike. At high levels of competency, the practitioner learns to redirect an aggressor's negative *Ki* during an attack thus causing it to betray him in the process.

Breath Control: Taekwondo requires that the body act in accordance with itself by synchronizing the breath to a particular action. This adds power, efficiency, and mindful intent to self-defense training. Just as a conductor leads a symphony orchestra, so the breath, acting in concert with *Ki,* balance, and momentum, must take control by adding explosive force to a strike on impact. For the most part, this is accomplished through the *kihop* or spirit yell. By exhaling the breath forcefully from *tanjun,* a focal point for *Ki* two inches below the navel, the practitioner will add power and purpose to a strike or block. Conversely, holding the breath while striking or blocking will ultimately restrict the effectiveness of the technique resulting in a substantial reduction of power.

Counterattacking: Since Gichin Funakoshi, founder of Shotokan karate, established that it is a prime responsibility of the martial artist not to initiate an attack by his statement, "there is no first attack in karate," counterattacking then is the essence of the art of self-defense. The practice of *il su sik, ho sin sool,* and other standard methods of training, sharpen the reflexes to the point where the practitioner can almost sense an incoming technique before it is executed. If a block is delivered with intent and purpose, it can have the equal effect of almost any strike. In our *dojang* it is taught "that a block is a strike." Often a well-placed counterattack will end a confrontation early on, precluding the necessity for further physical contact with the attacker. This is no small consideration in a world of blood-borne diseases. Furthermore, since a block is potentially less damaging than a hard, linear technique such as a palm heel strike (*batang son chilki*), reverse punch (*bandae jiluki*), or round kick (*dollyo chagi*), given the severity of a situation, it may be in the best interest of the defender to terminate a dispute with a technique of this nature. Either way, counterattacking lies at the defensive core of martial arts training and developing the ability to respond swiftly is essential.

Technical Proficiency: It is a given fact that if one practices diligently and with sincerity, technical proficiency will increase. This process will be augmented if *il su sik* and *ho sin sool* techniques are taught in ever diminishing circles. At successive levels, the student should first be exposed to the gross motions of a predetermined defensive tactic. Subsequently, with each practice session, the combination is increasingly refined and distilled down in greater detail. A pedagogical approach of this nature reveals the practical application of the various elements that compose a unique combination while allowing the individual techniques to segue freely from one to the other. As skill in the technique increases, the student will further the quality of the combination by successfully activating various acupoints on the body thus supporting the effectiveness of the technique. This can only be accomplished through a high degree of practice.

Coordination: Coordination is developed in taekwondo regardless of the area of concentration. Basics, *poom-se*, kicking, and self-defense drills all require that various parts of the body act in harmony while performing dissimilar actions. Often, one hand may be blocking while the opposite foot is kicking causing the newcomer to feel extremely challenged and left wondering if technique will ever be executed in concert. Surprisingly, after only a few classes, even the most ungainly person begins to show a marked improvement in the management of body mechanics. For an instructor, it is very rewarding to observe the pupil progress from a chaotic jumble of hands and feet to an effectively coordinated defensive machine. Likewise, for the student, the ability to move with fluidity while executing multiple techniques in chorus is a sure sign of progress.

While most of the above considerations are specific to the martial arts, others are clearly of the sort one would ordinarily not associate with the practice of self-defense. It should be noted, however, that traditional taekwondo is, above all, a holistic pursuit and therefore not limited merely to physical technique. One cannot overemphasize the importance of respect when practicing a potentially lethal art. By the same token, all the courtesy in the world will not come to one's aid when set upon by a willful aggressor resulting in the development of collateral skills by the sincere practitioner. However, as we have seen in previous sections of this book, various tools exist that support the ritualized practice of il su sik and ho sin sool by helping to organize the body and spirit into a mindful source of focused energy prepared to provide self-protection.

CHAPTER 9

Il Su Sik Practice

The defensive tactics that follow, progress from relatively simple combinations of techniques, to strategies that require a pronounced level of proficiency. As always, it is wise to begin slowly and master each motion before moving on to the next. Moreover, in attempting to perform these highly effective and elegant self-defense sequences, one must remember to proceed with great caution as well as purpose. Once mastered, however, the martial artist will find them extremely useful as additional tools in their arsenal of traditional taekwondo skills.

Emphasis should be placed on several key elements during the practice of *il su sik* and *sam su sik.**

- Always use caution during practice.
- Practice slow and deliberately in the beginning.
- Approach the application of these techniques with utmost seriousness as though you were truly being attacked.
- These techniques must become ingrained if they are to be effective.
- Always bow at the beginning of self-defense training to display respect and courtesy.
- *Kihop* vigorously at the appointed times to demonstrate intent and to motivate your training partner.
- Check your distance before commencing in an effort to make your practice more effective and meaningful.
- Maintain proper stances throughout the sequence.
- Concentrate and maintain focus.
- Practice both the left and right sides of the body.
- Blocks should remain within the body margin.
- Commit the initial block before executing an appropriate counterattack.
- Students are encouraged to experiment and create defensive sequences of their own within the bounds of traditional taekwondo technique.
- One- and three-step sparring practice is not limited to self-defense against punches, but can also include counterattacks against kicking techniques.

*The practice drills for sam su sik begin in Chapter 10

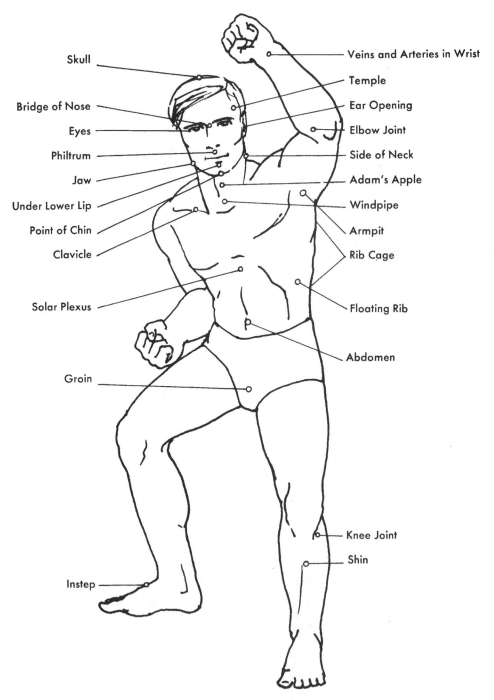

Skull

Bridge of Nose

Eyes

Philtrum

Jaw

Under Lower Lip

Point of Chin

Clavicle

Solar Plexus

Groin

Instep

Veins and Arteries in Wrist

Temple

Ear Opening

Elbow Joint

Side of Neck

Adam's Apple

Windpipe

Armpit

Rib Cage

Floating Rib

Abdomen

Knee Joint

Shin

Vital Points (front).

From Chun, Richard. Taekwondo: A Korean Martial Art
New York, Harper & Row, 1976.

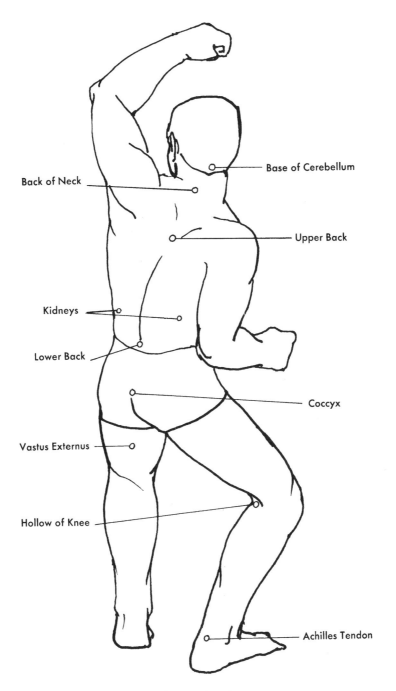

Base of Cerebellum

Back of Neck

Upper Back

Kidneys

Lower Back

Coccyx

Vastus Externus

Hollow of Knee

Achilles Tendon

From Chun, Richard. *Taekwondo: A Korean Martial Art* New York, Harper & Row, 1976.

Vital Points (rear).

Il Su Sik Drills—Il Su Sik 1

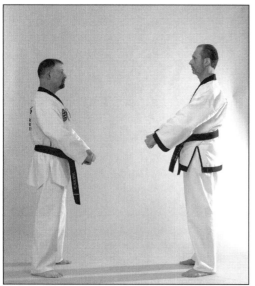

a. *Joombi* position.

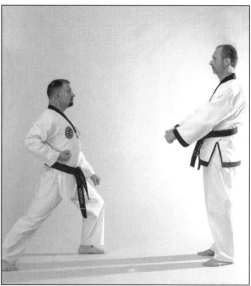

b. Attacker slides right foot back assuming a left front stance while performing a left low block.

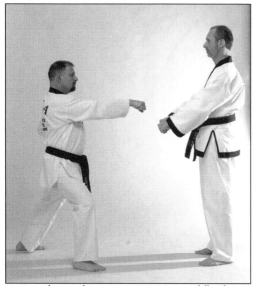

c. Attacker advances executing middle lunge punch in front stance.

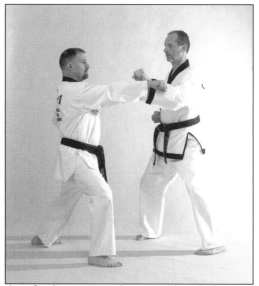

d. Defender steps 45 degrees with right foot into horse stance while simultaneously performing a left hand in/out middle block.

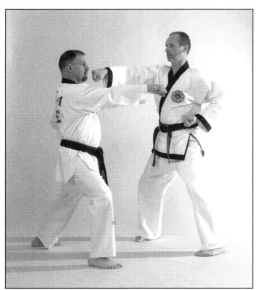

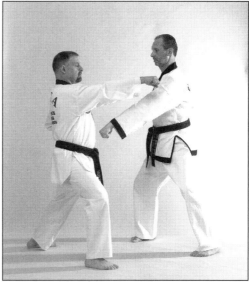

e. Immediately execute a right hand high punch to the face.

f. Finish with a left hand middle punch to the solar plexus.

IL SU SIK 2

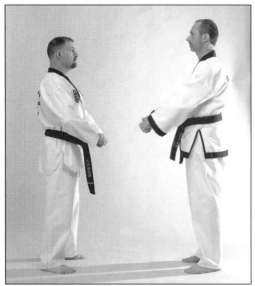

a. *Joombi* position.

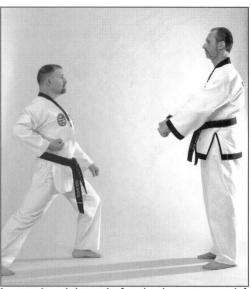

b. Attacker slides right foot back assuming a left front stance while performing a left low block.

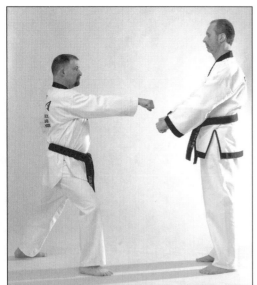

c. Attacker advances executing middle lunge punch in front stance.

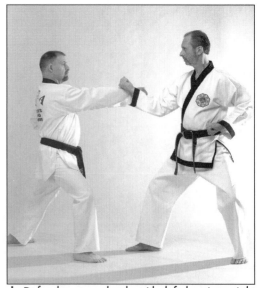

d. Defender steps back with left leg into right back stance while executing right hand in/out middle block.

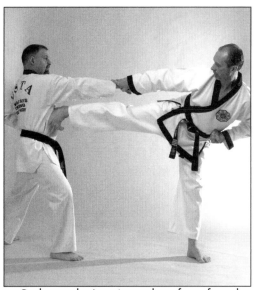 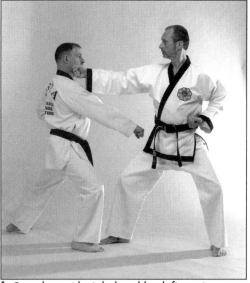

e. Grab attacker's wrist and perform front leg side kick to ribs.

f. Complete with right hand back fist to jaw.

Il Su Sik 3

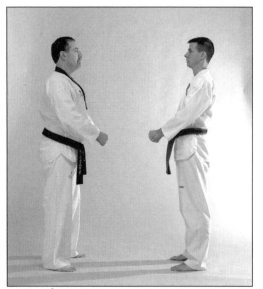

a. *Joombi* position.

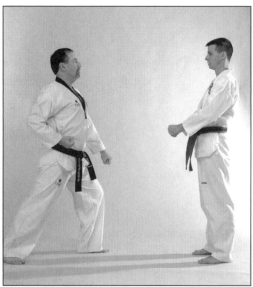

b. Attacker slides right foot back assuming a left front stance while.

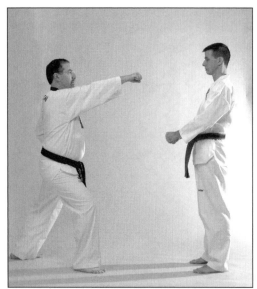

c. Attacker advances executing high punch in front stance.

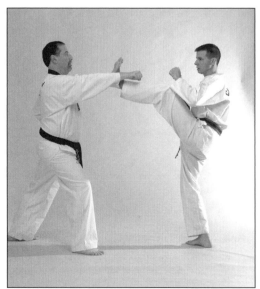

d. Defender redirects strike with a left leg in/out crescent kick.

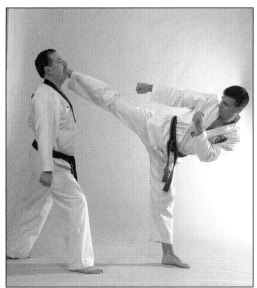

e. Complete with a right-leg round kick to the face.

Il Su Sik 4

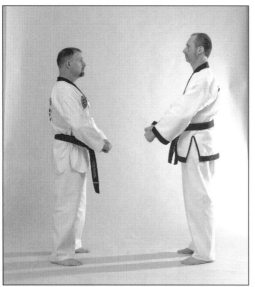

a. *Joombi* position.

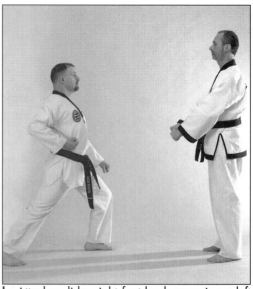

b. Attacker slides right foot back assuming a left front stance while performing a left low block.

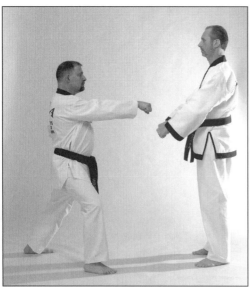

c. Attacker advances executing middle lunge punch in front stance.

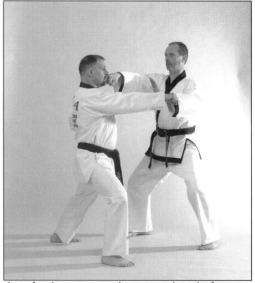

d. Defender steps 45 degrees with right foot into horse stance while simultaneously performing a left hand in/out middle knife block and high punch to face.

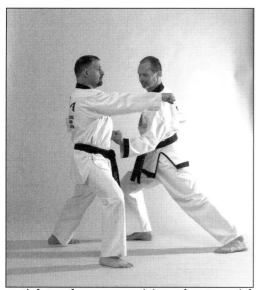

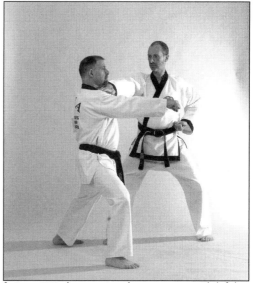

e. Shift into front stance while performing a left hand upper cut to opponent's solar plexus.

f. Step 270 degrees into horse stance with left leg while pivoting on the ball of the right foot and complete with a right hand knife strike to attacker's throat.

Il Su Sik 5

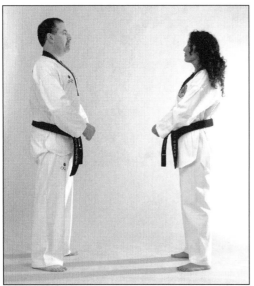

a. *Joombi* position.

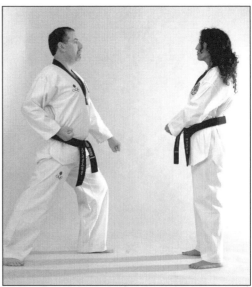

b. Attacker slides right foot back assuming a left front stance while performing a left low block.

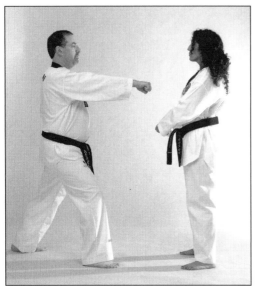

c. Attacker advances executing middle lunge punch in front stance.

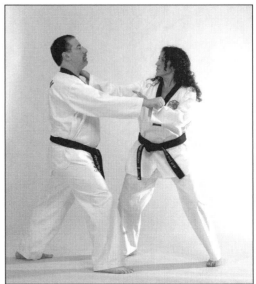

d. Defender steps 45 degrees with right foot into horse stance while simultaneously performing a left hand in/out middle knife block and right hand knife strike to side of opponent's neck.

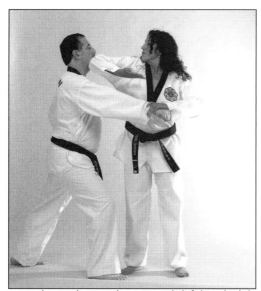

e. Grab attacker's right wrist with left hand while sliding right leg back into upright stance. Complete with right side elbow strike to temple.

IL SU SIK 6

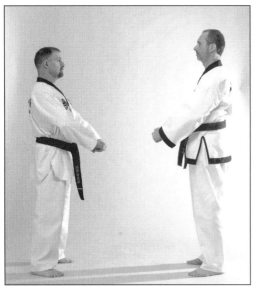

a. *Joombi* position.

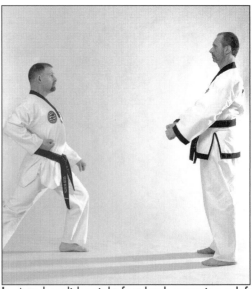

b. Attacker slides right foot back assuming a left front stance while performing a left low block.

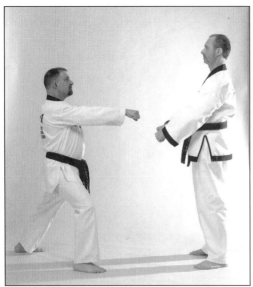

c. Attacker advances executing middle lunge punch in front stance.

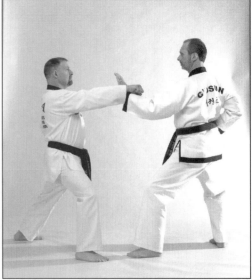

d. Defender steps back with right leg into left back stance while performing a left hand in/out middle knife block.

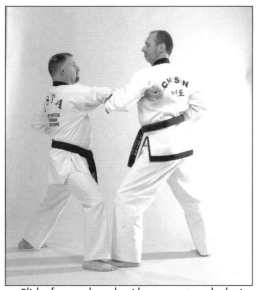

e. Slide forward and with a counter clockwise motion, execute a left arm bar.

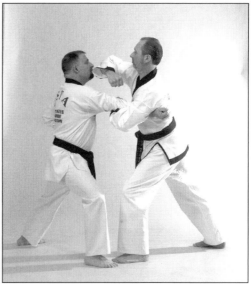

f. Execute a right round elbow strike to face.

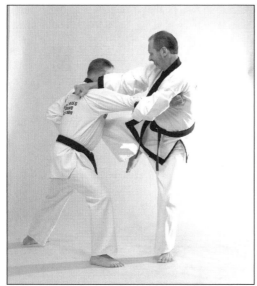

g. Grasp attacker's right shoulder with right hand and complete with right round knee strike to solar plexus.

Il Su Sik 7

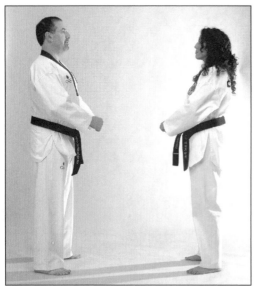

a. *Joombi* position.

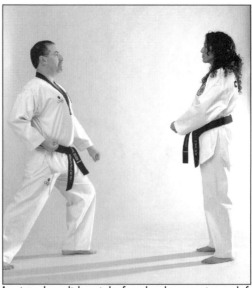

b. Attacker slides right foot back assuming a left front stance while performing a left low block.

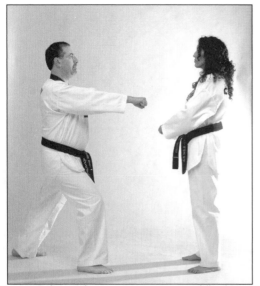

c. Attacker advances executing middle lunge punch in front stance.

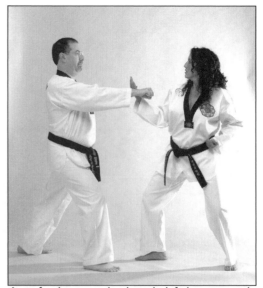

d. Defender steps back with left leg into right back stance while performing right hand out/in middle knife block.

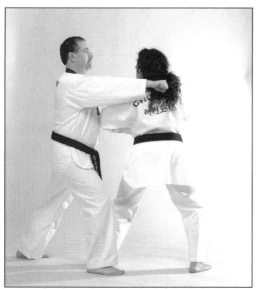

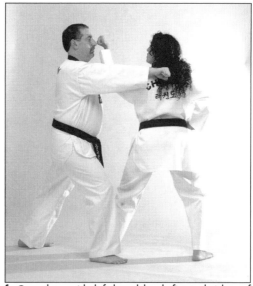

e. Pivot backwards and to the left 180 degrees on the right foot into horse stance while executing left side elbow strike to ribs.

f. Complete with left hand back fist to bridge of nose.

Il Su Sik 8

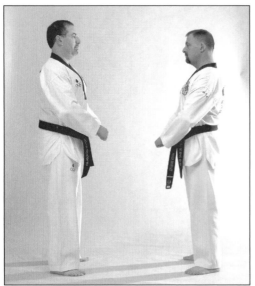

a. *Joombi* position.

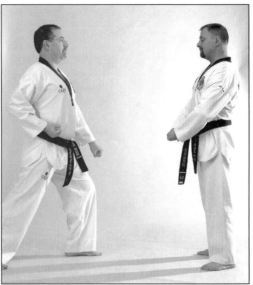

b. Attacker slides right foot back assuming a left front stance while performing a left low block.

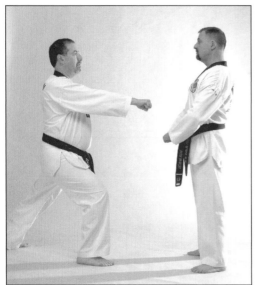

c. Attacker advances executing middle lunge punch in front stance.

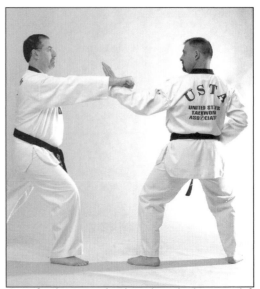

d. Defender steps back with right leg into left back stance while performing left hand in/out middle knife block.

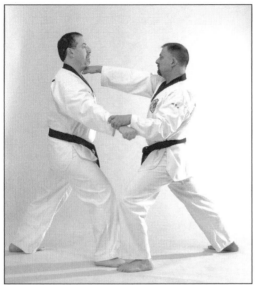

e. Quickly grab attacker's right wrist and shift into front stance while executing right hand tiger mouth strike to throat.

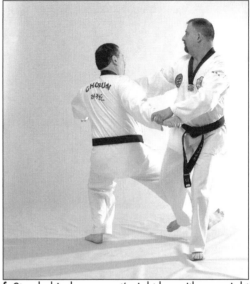

f. Step behind opponent's right leg with your right foot and sweep to ground.

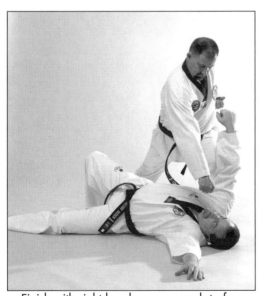

g. Finish with right hand reverse punch to face.

Il Su Sik 9

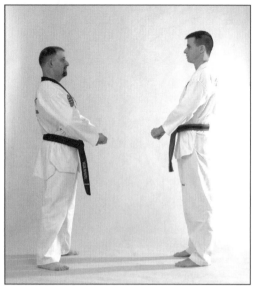

a. *Joombi* position.

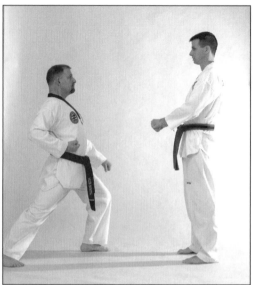

b. Attacker slides right foot back assuming a left front stance while performing a left low block.

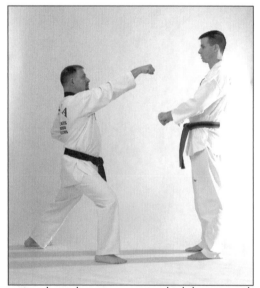

c. Attacker advances executing high lunge punch in front stance.

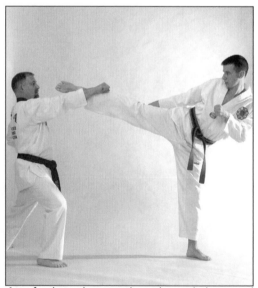

d. Defender redirects strike with a right leg round kick to the arm.

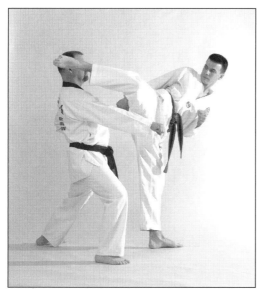

e. After return kicking foot to the ground, finish with a right-leg hop step hook kick to the face.

Il Su Sik 10

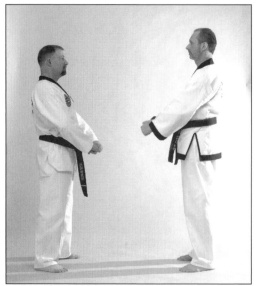

a. *Joombi* position.

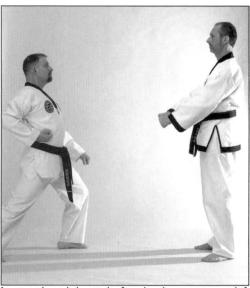

b. Attacker slides right foot back assuming a left front stance while performing a left low block.

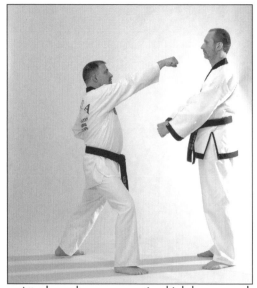

c. Attacker advances executing high lunge punch in front stance.

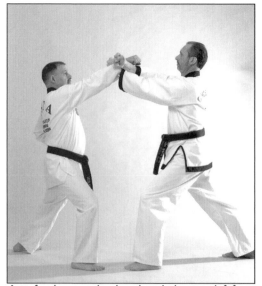

d. Defender steps back with right leg into left front stance while performing a high X block.

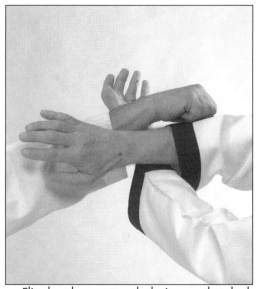

e. Flip hands counter clockwise so that both palms are facing inward.

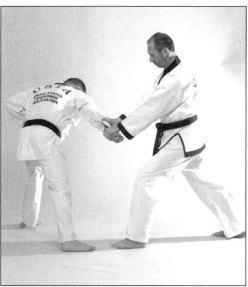

f. Grab attacker's wrist and twist in a downward, clockwise motion.

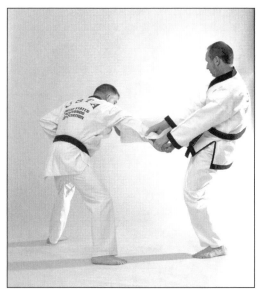

g. Execute a front kick to face.

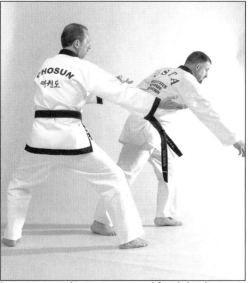

h. Step into a horse stance and finish by throwing opponent to your right.

IL SU SIK 11

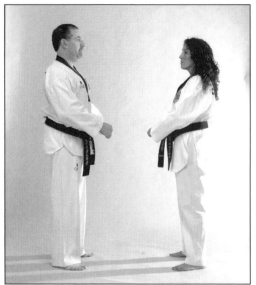

a. *Joombi* position.

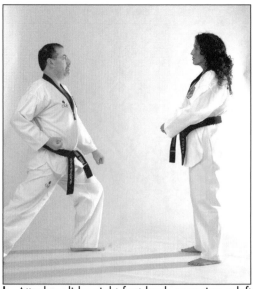

b. Attacker slides right foot back assuming a left front stance while performing a left low block.

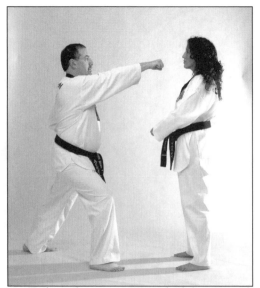

c. Attacker advances executing high lunge punch in front stance.

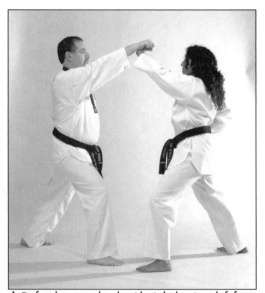

d. Defender steps back with right leg into left front stance while performing a left hand high block.

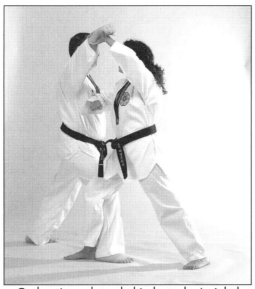

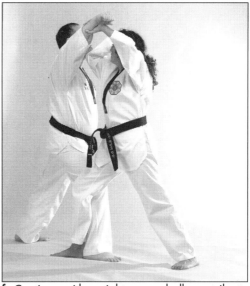

e. Grab wrist and step behind attacker's right leg with your right foot while executing a round elbow strike to solar plexus.

f. Continue with a right upward elbow strike to chin.

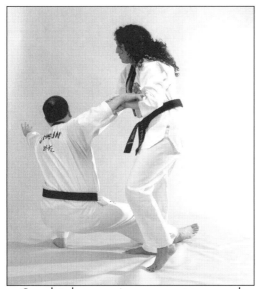

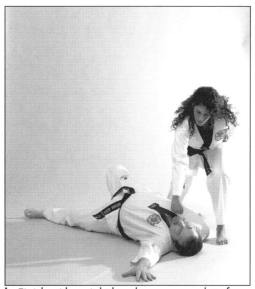

g. Complete by sweeping opponent to ground.

h. Finish with a right hand reverse punch to face.

Il Su Sik 12

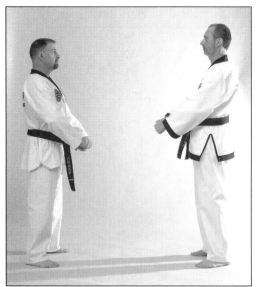

a. *Joombi* position.

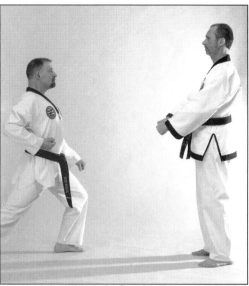

b. Attacker slides right foot back assuming a left front stance while performing a left low block.

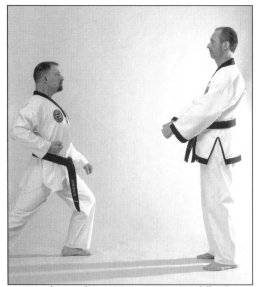

c. Attacker advances executing middle lunge punch in front stance.

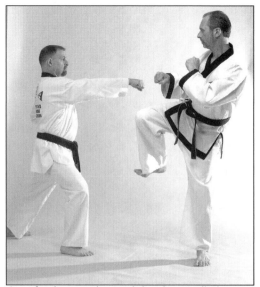

d. Defender avoids attack by diagonally leaping one step to the left, bringing weight down on the left foot only.

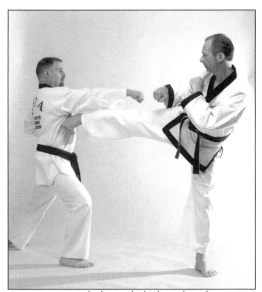

e. Execute a right leg side kick to the ribs.

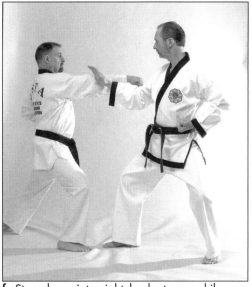

f. Step down into right back stance while performing right hand in/out knife strike to opponent's right elbow.

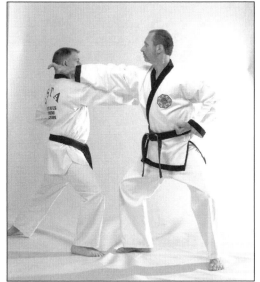

g. Finish with right hand in/out knife strike to side of neck.

Il Su Sik 13

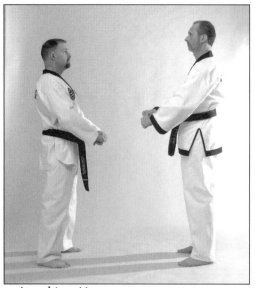

a. *Joombi* position.

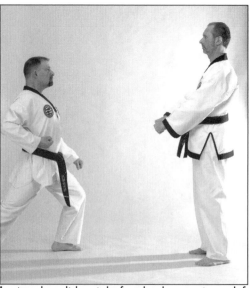

b. Attacker slides right foot back assuming a left front stance while performing a left low block.

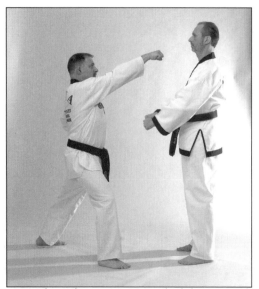

c. Attacker advances executing high lunge punch in front stance.

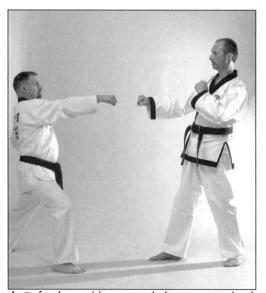

d. Defender yields to punch by stepping back with left leg into left fighting stance.

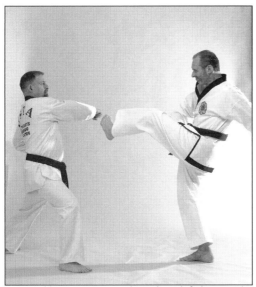

e. Quickly counter punch with a left leg out/in crescent kick.

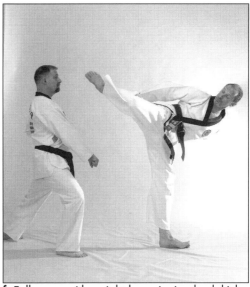

f. Follow up with a right leg spinning hook kick.

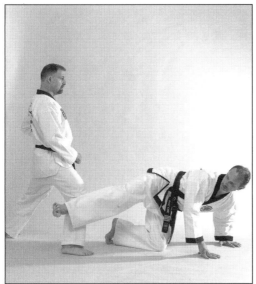

g. Dropping on your left knee and the palms of both hands, force attacker to the ground with a right leg spinning sweep kick.

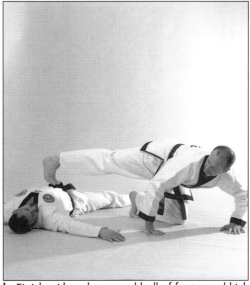

h. Finish with a downward ball of foot round kick to the solar plexus.

Il Su Sik 14

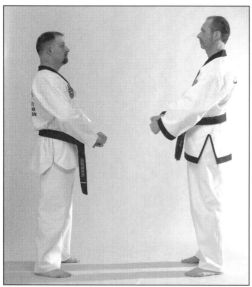

a. *Joombi* position.

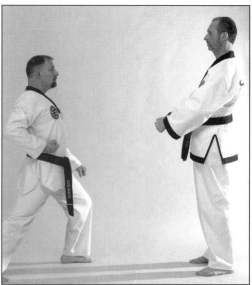

b. Attacker slides right foot back assuming a left front stance while performing a left low block.

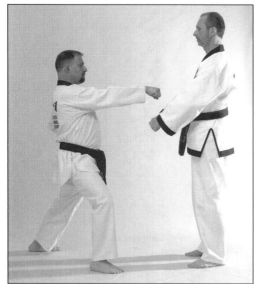

c. Attacker advances executing middle lunge punch in front stance.

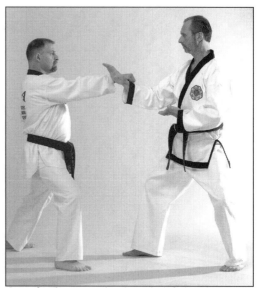

d. Defender steps back with left leg into right back stance while performing double hand in/out middle knife block.

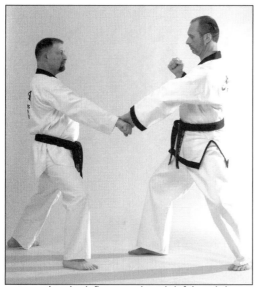

e. Immediately deflect punch with left hand downward palm heel block.

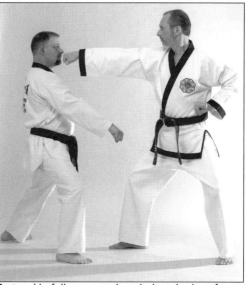

f. Quickly follow up with right hand jab to face.

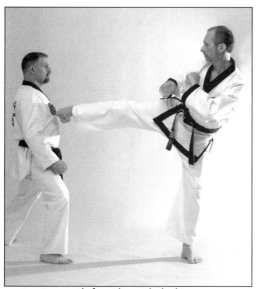

g. Continue with front leg side kick.

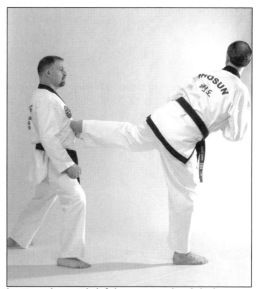

h. Complete with left leg turning back kick.

Il Su Sik 15

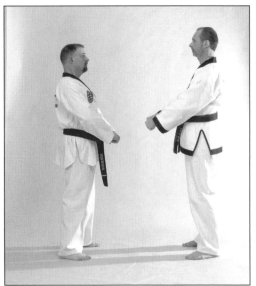

a. *Joombi* position.

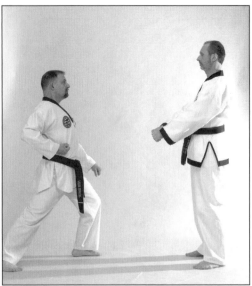

b. Attacker slides right foot back assuming a left front stance while performing a left low block.

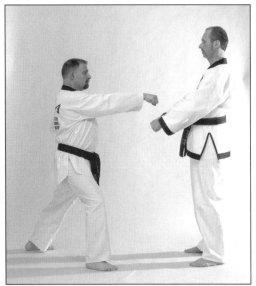

c. Attacker advances executing middle lunge punch in front stance.

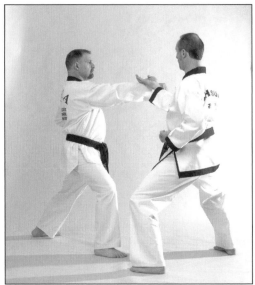

d. Defender steps 45 degrees with left foot into horse stance while simultaneously performing a right in/out middle ridge hand block, palm up.

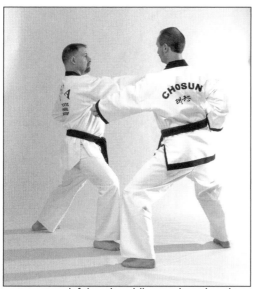

e. Execute a left hand middle punch to the ribs.

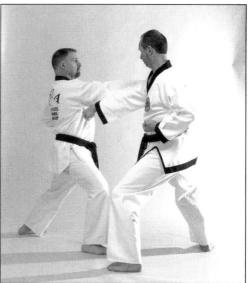

f. Immediately follow up with a right hand middle punch to the ribs.

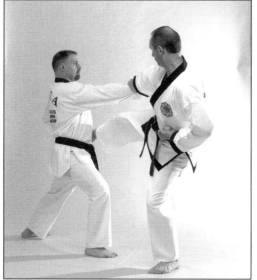

g. Grab attacker's right wrist with your right hand and execute a right leg round kick to the solar plexus.

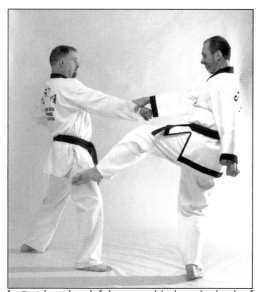

h. Finish with a left leg round kick to the back of opponent's thigh.

Il Su Sik 16

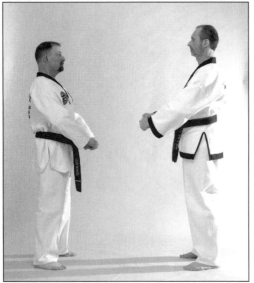

a. *Joombi* position.

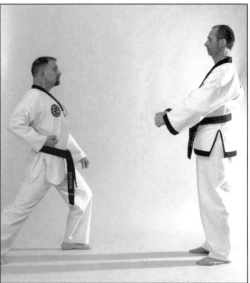

b. Attacker slides right foot back assuming a left front stance while performing a left low block.

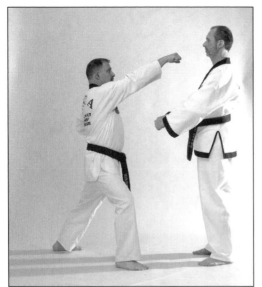

c. Attacker advances executing high lunge punch in front stance.

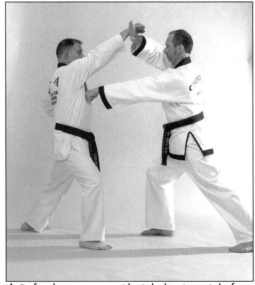

d. Defender steps up with right leg into right front stance while simultaneously executing a right hand high knife block and left hand middle punch to the attacker's solar plexus.

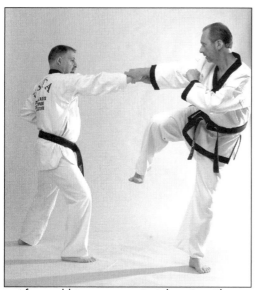

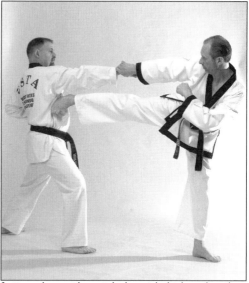

e. After grabbing opponent's right wrist with your right hand, step to the left.

f. Complete with a right leg side kick to the ribs.

Il Su Sik 17

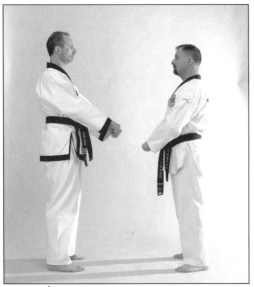

a. *Joombi* position.

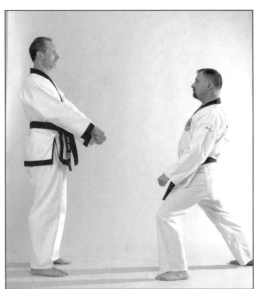

b. Attacker slides right foot back assuming a left front stance while performing a left low block.

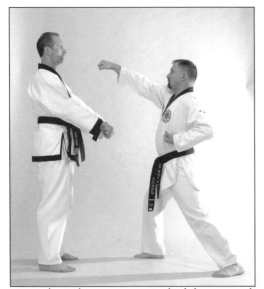

c. Attacker advances executing high lunge punch in front stance.

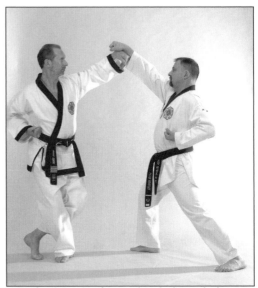

d. Defender steps forward with the right leg into twist stance while performing a left hand ox jaw block.

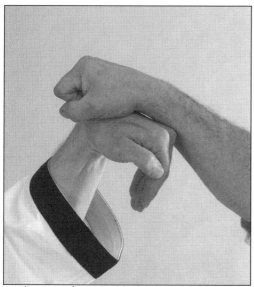

e. Close up of ox jaw block.

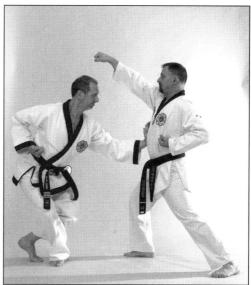

f. Quickly follow up with a left downward palm heel strike to the opponent's ribs.

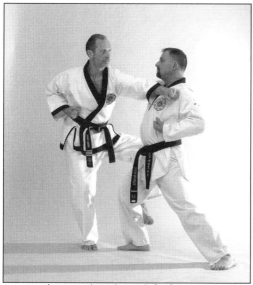

g. Simultaneously place left forearm across attacker's upper chest and the sole of your left foot behind the knee.

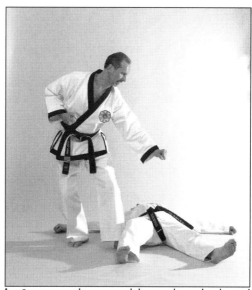

h. Sweep to the ground by pushing backward with your arm and forward with your foot.

IL SU SIK 17 *(CONTINUED)*

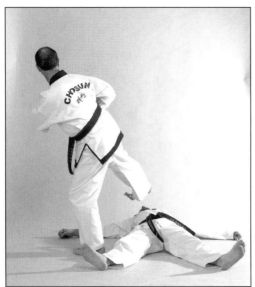

i. Turning slightly to your right, finish by executing a downward side kick to opponent's face.

IL SU SIK 18

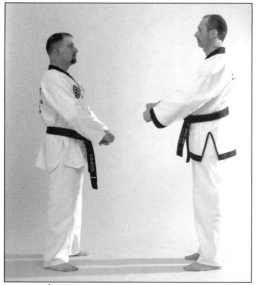

a. *Joombi* position.

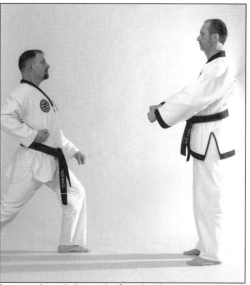

b. Attacker slides right foot back assuming a left front stance while performing a left low block.

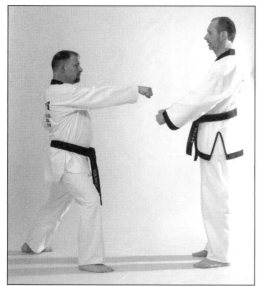

c. Attacker advances executing middle lunge punch in front stance.

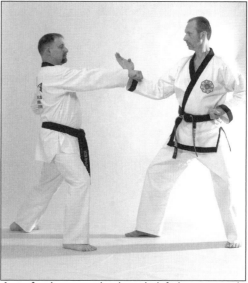

d. Defender steps back with left leg into right back stance while performing right hand out/in middle knife block.

IL SU SIK 18 (CONTINUED)

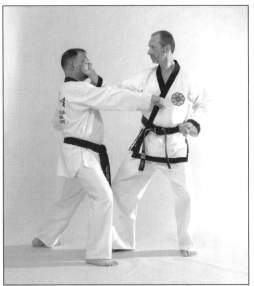

e. Slide one step towards attacker and deliver a downward right hand back fist to bridge of nose.

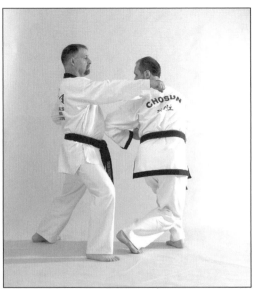

f. Pivot 180 degrees to your left coming up on the ball of the right foot while executing a left elbow strike to opponent's solar plexus.

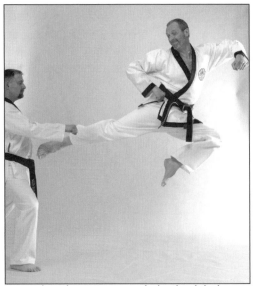

g. Finish with a jumping right-leg back kick.

CHAPTER 10
Sam Su Sik Practice

For principles of *sam su sik* practice, refer to Chapter 9.

SAM SU SIK DRILLS—*SAM SU SIK* 1

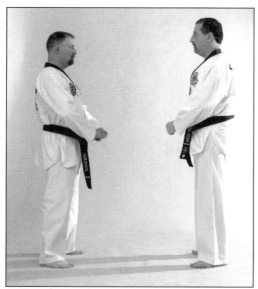

a. *Joombi* position.

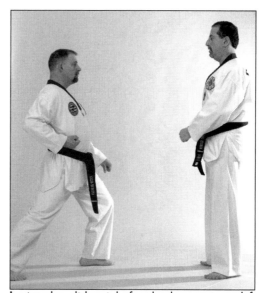

b. Attacker slides right foot back assuming a left front stance while performing a left low block.

SAM SU SIK 1 *(CONTINUED)*

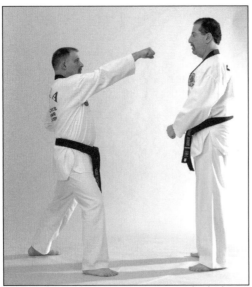

c. Attacker advances executing a high lunge punch in right front stance.

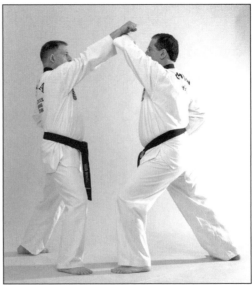

d. Defender steps back with right leg into a left front stance while executing a left high block in response to high punch.

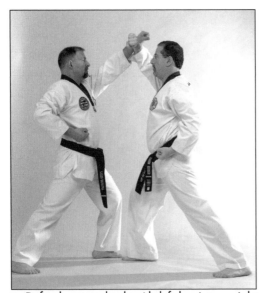

e. Defender steps back with left leg into a right front stance while executing a right high block in response to high punch.

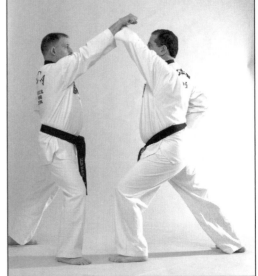

f. Defender steps back with right leg into a left front stance while executing a left high block in response to high punch.

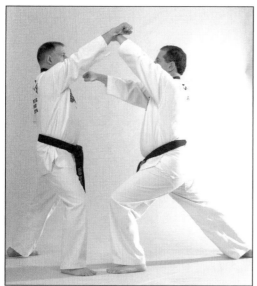

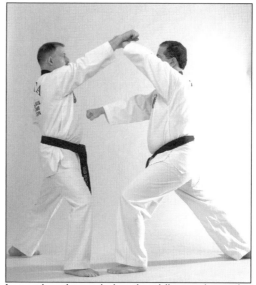

g. While maintaining the front stance and high block, defender counterattacks with a right hand high punch to face.

h. Finish with a right hand middle punch to solar plexus.

SAM SU SIK 2

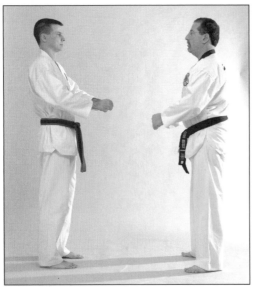

a. *Joombi* position.

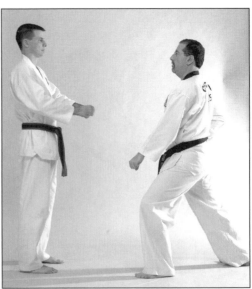

b. Attacker slides right foot back assuming a left front stance while performing a left low block.

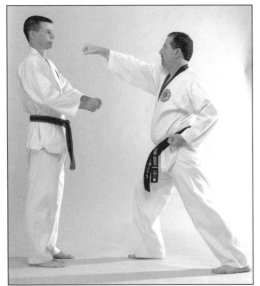

c. Attacker advances executing a high lunge punch in right front stance.

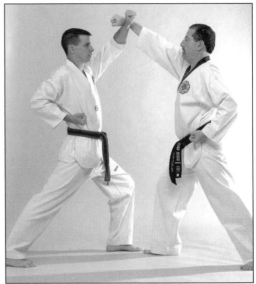

d. Defender steps back with right leg into a left front stance while executing a left high block in response to high punch.

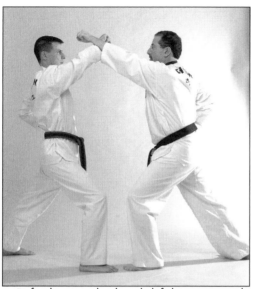

e. Defender steps back with left leg into a right front stance while executing a right high block in response to high punch.

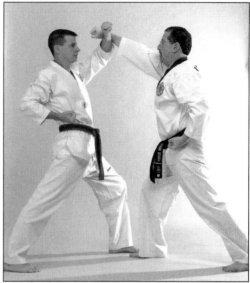

f. Defender steps back with right leg into a left front stance while executing a left high block in response to high punch.

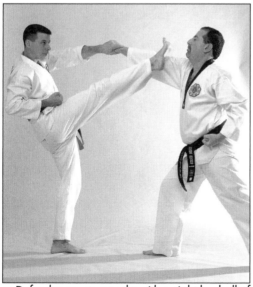

g. Defender counterattacks with a right leg ball of foot front kick to face.

SAM SU SIK 3

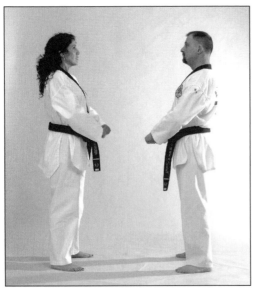

a. *Joombi* position.

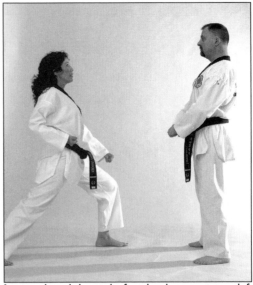

b. Attacker slides right foot back assuming a left front stance while performing a left low block.

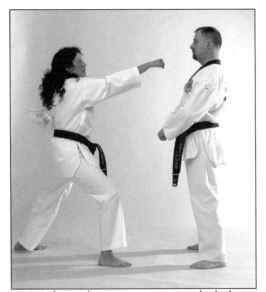

c. Attacker advances executing a high lunge punch in right front stance.

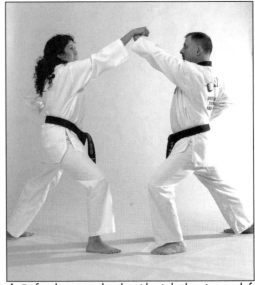

d. Defender steps back with right leg into a left front stance while executing a left high block in response to high punch.

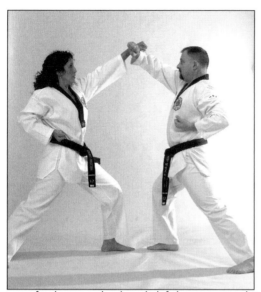

e. Defender steps back with left leg into a right front stance while executing a right high block in response to high punch.

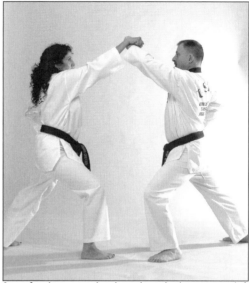

f. Defender steps back with right leg into a left front stance while executing a left high block in response to high punch.

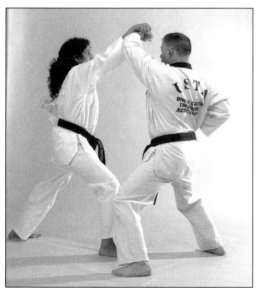

g. While maintaining the high block, defender slides 45 degrees to the attacker's right into horse stance.

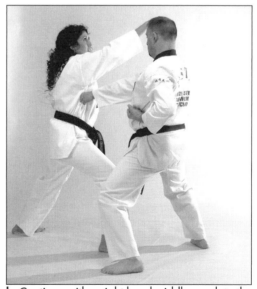

h. Continue with a right hand middle punch to the ribs.

SAM SU SIK 3 (CONTINUED)

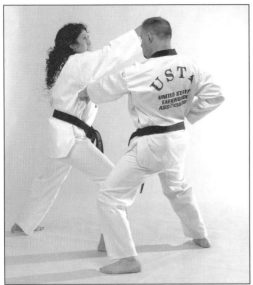

i. Finish with a left hand middle punch to the ribs.

SAM SU SIK 4

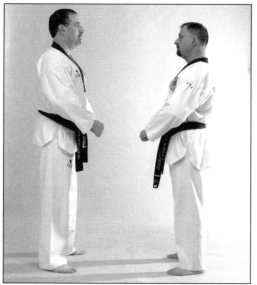

a. *Joombi* position.

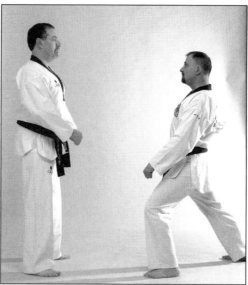

b. Attacker slides right foot back assuming a left front stance while performing a left low block.

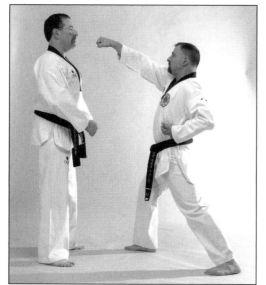

c. Attacker advances executing a high lunge punch in right front stance.

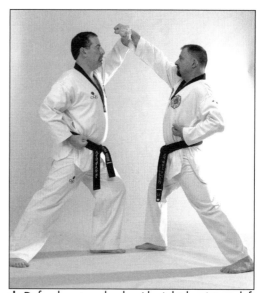

d. Defender steps back with right leg into a left front stance while executing a left high block in response to high punch.

SAM SU SIK 4 (CONTINUED)

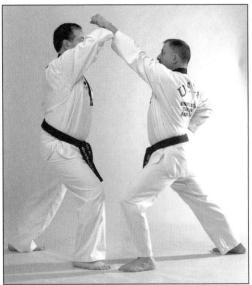

e. Defender steps back with left leg into a right front stance while executing a right high block in response to high punch.

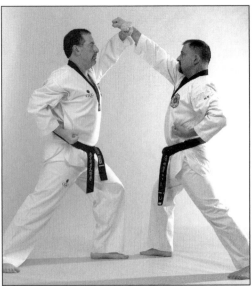

f. Defender steps back with right leg into a left front stance while executing a left high block in response to high punch.

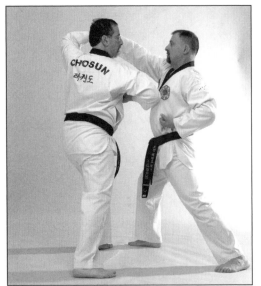

g. Defender steps 45 degrees to the attacker's left assuming horse stance while executing a right round elbow strike to the solar plexus.

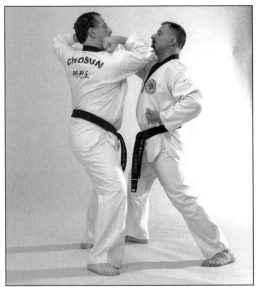

h. Complete with a right upward elbow strike to the chin.

SAM SU SIK 5

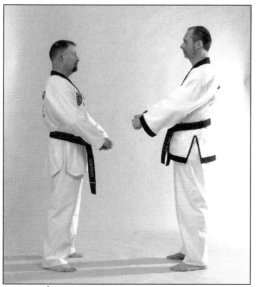

a. *Joombi* position.

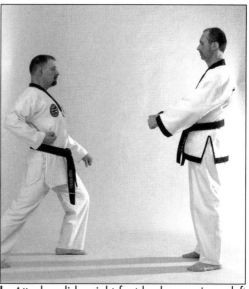

b. Attacker slides right foot back assuming a left front stance while performing a left low block.

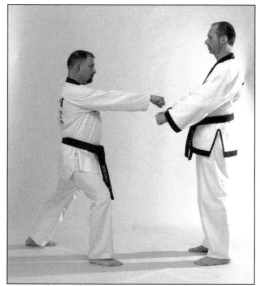

c. Attacker advances executing a middle lunge punch in right front stance.

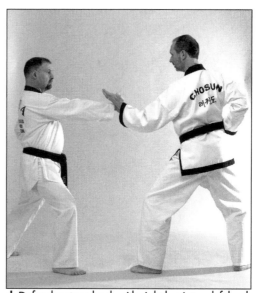

d. Defender steps back with right leg into a left back stance while executing a left hand out/in knife block to the outside of the opponent's right arm.

SAM SU SIK 5 (CONTINUED)

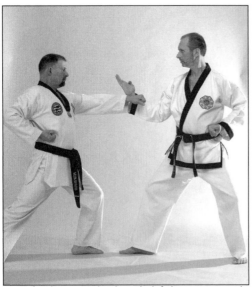

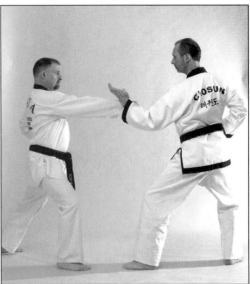

e. Defender steps back with left leg into a right back stance while executing a right hand out/in knife block to the outside of the opponent's left arm.

f. Defender steps back with right leg into a left back stance while executing a left hand out/in knife block to the outside of the opponent's right arm.

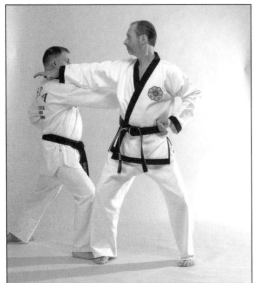

g. Defender counterattacks by stepping 180 degrees to the right into horse stance and executing a right hand knife strike to the opponent's neck.

SAM SU SIK 6

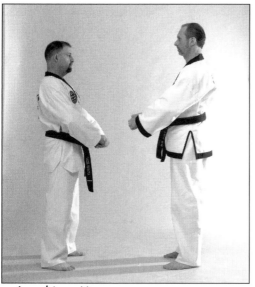

a. *Joombi* position.

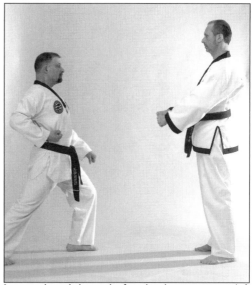

b. Attacker slides right foot back assuming a left front stance while performing a left low block.

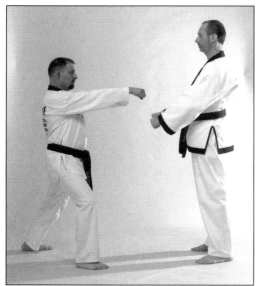

c. Attacker advances executing a middle lunge punch in right front stance.

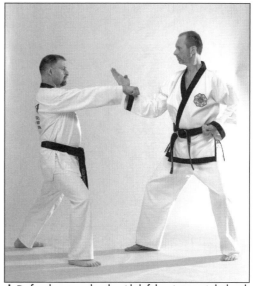

d. Defender steps back with left leg into a right back stance while executing a right hand out/in knife block to the inside of the opponent's right arm.

SAM SU SIK 6 (CONTINUED)

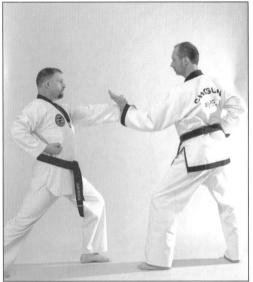

e. Defender steps back with right leg into a left back stance while executing a left hand out/in knife block to the inside of the opponent's left arm.

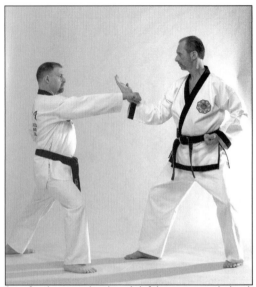

f. Defender steps back with left leg into a right back stance while executing a right hand out/in knife block to the inside of the opponent's right arm.

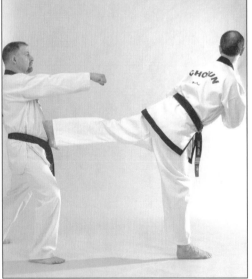

g. Defender counterattacks by executing a turning back kick with the left leg to attacker's solar plexus.

SAM SU SIK 7

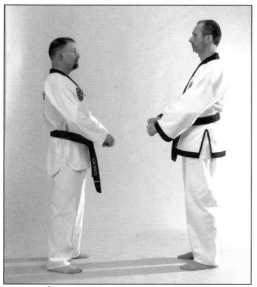

a. *Joombi* position.

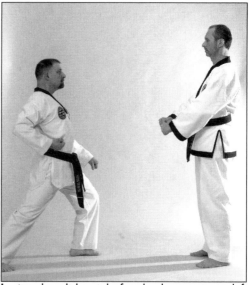

b. Attacker slides right foot back assuming a left front stance while performing a left low block.

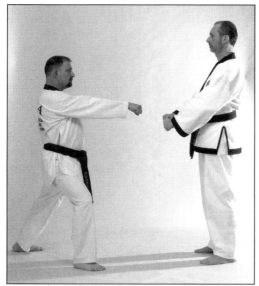

c. Attacker advances executing a middle lunge punch in right front stance.

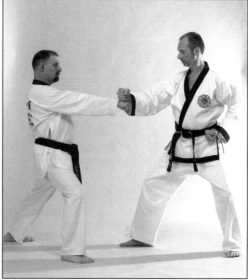

d. Defender steps back with left leg into a right back stance while executing a right hand downward hammer fist to opponent's right wrist.

SAM SU SIK 7 *(CONTINUED)*

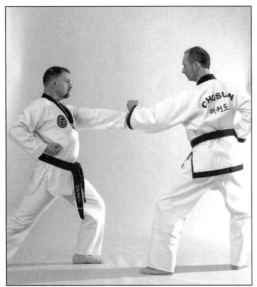

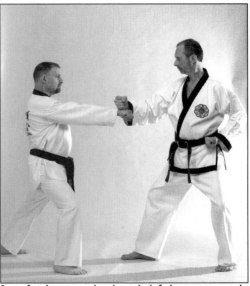

e. Defender steps back with right leg into a left back stance while executing a left hand downward hammer fist to opponent's left wrist.

f. Defender steps back with left leg into a right back stance while executing a right hand downward hammer fist to opponent's right wrist.

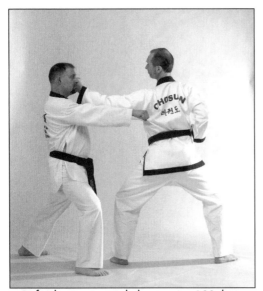

g. Defender counterattacks by stepping 180 degrees to the left into horse stance and executing a left hand spinning back fist to the opponent's head.

SAM SU SIK 8

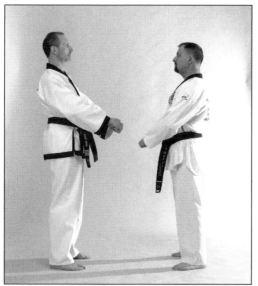

a. *Joombi* position.

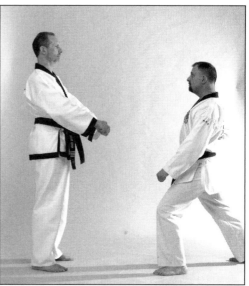

b. Attacker slides right foot back assuming a left front stance while performing a left low block.

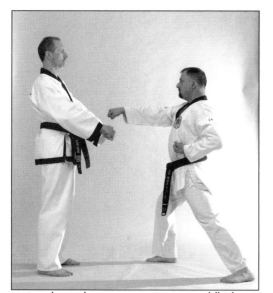

c. Attacker advances executing a middle lunge punch in right front stance.

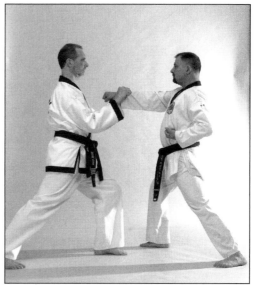

d. Defender steps back with right leg into a left front stance while executing a double spread block to opponent's right wrist.

SAM SU SIK 8 (CONTINUED)

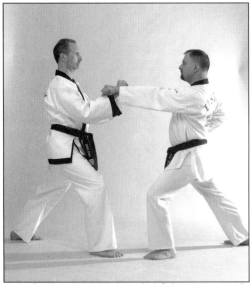

e. Defender steps back with left leg into a right front stance while executing a double spread block to opponent's left wrist.

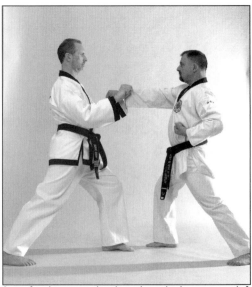

f. Defender steps back with right leg into a left front stance while executing a double spread block to opponent's right wrist.

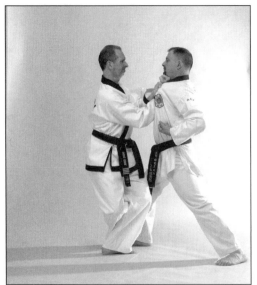

g. Defender steps into twist stance with right leg and counterattacks by grabbing opponent's shirt with left hand while executing a right hand upper cut to chin.

CHAPTER 11
Ho Sin Sool Practice

The techniques illustrated below, both simple and complex, are not exclusive to traditional taekwondo but borrow also from hapkido, aikido and, to some extent, judo. They have been chosen for this book, however, for their simplicity and ease of use; two crucial elements of practical self-defense. For illustrative purposes, the attacker is grabbing in most cases with the right hand. This is because a great majority of people are right-handed. Regardless, these techniques will work on either side of the body and should be practiced accordingly. During the initial practice of these traditional defensive strategies a number of cautionary measures should be followed, which you will find echoed later in the principles of women's self-defense:

- Always use caution during practice.
- Do not develop a "false sense of security."
- Practice slowly and deliberately in the beginning.
- Approach the application of these techniques with utmost seriousness as though you were truly being attacked.
- These techniques must become ingrained if they are to be effective.
- Remember to have attacking partner "tap out" in response to an effective technique.

Finally, it is wise to use a technique to the point of submission, then escape. Remember: the ultimate goal of self-defense is to escape unharmed, not simply to injure your attacker.

HO SIN SOOL DRILLS—HO SIN SOOL 1

(Defense against same side grab)

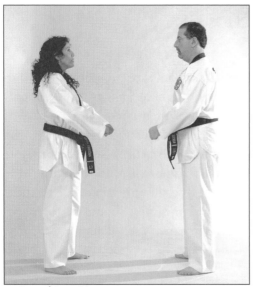

a. *Joombi* position.

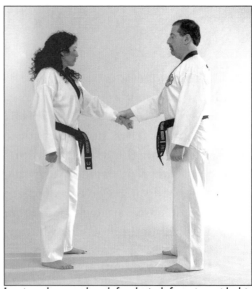

b. Attacker grabs defender's left wrist with his right hand.

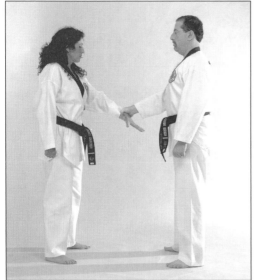

c. Defender spreads fingers, opening hand.

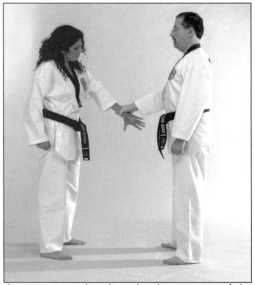

d. Rotate your hand so the thin portion of the wrist is facing the opening in the attacker's right.

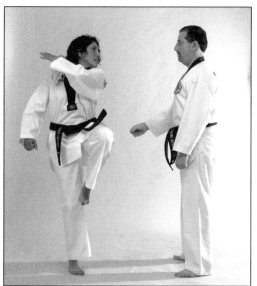

e. Force release by pulling wrist from attacker's grasp while simultaneously lifting left leg.

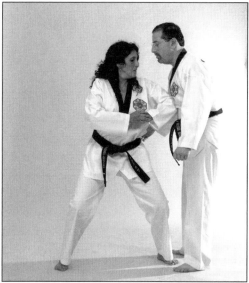

f. Step down into horse stance while executing a left elbow strike to opponent's solar plexus.

HO SIN SOOL 2

(Defense against same side grab)

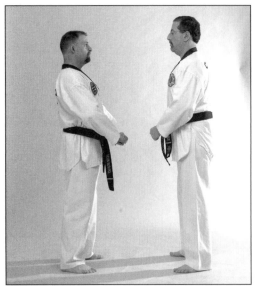

a. *Joombi* position.

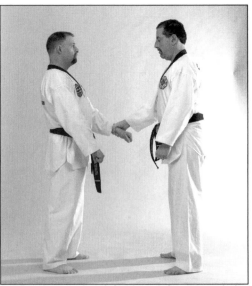

b. Attacker grabs defender's left wrist with his right hand.

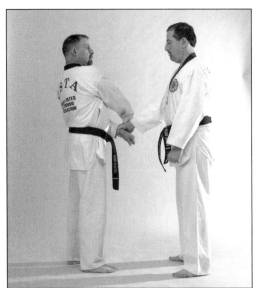

c. Reach over with your right hand gripping outside of attacker's hand while placing thumb on middle knuckle.

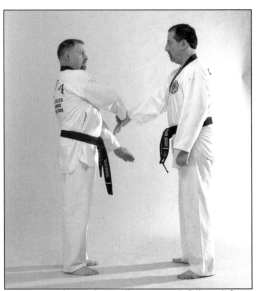

d. Force release by pulling your left hand from attacker's grasp.

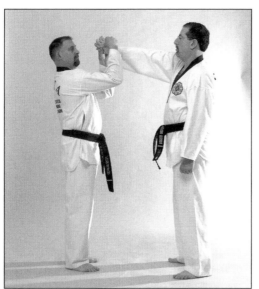

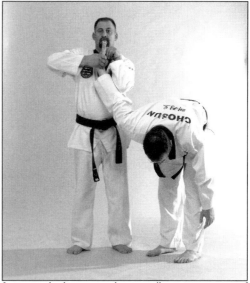

e. Once released, grab opponent's hand with your left, matching thumbs.

f. Twist clockwise until your elbow is on top of attacker's elbow and bear down, keeping opponent's hand level with your face.

HO SIN SOOL 3
(Defense against cross hand grab)

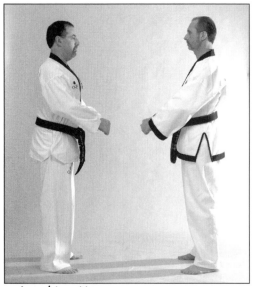

a. *Joombi* position.

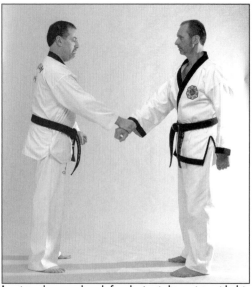

b. Attacker grabs defender's right wrist with his right hand.

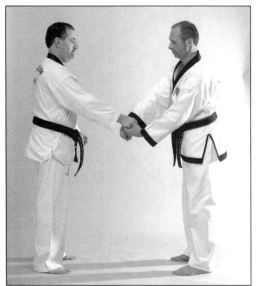

c. Grab attacker's right hand with your left placing thumb on middle knuckle.

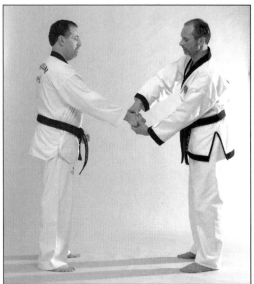

d. Release right hand and match thumbs.

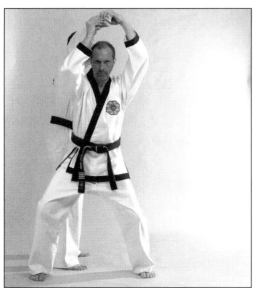

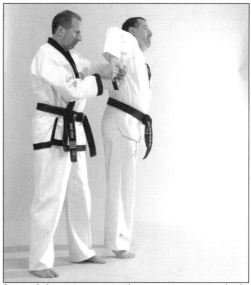

e. Step underneath opponent's right arm with your right leg.

f. Finish by twisting attacker's wrist counter clockwise while holding attacker's elbow high.

Ho Sin Sool 4

(Defense against cross hand grab)

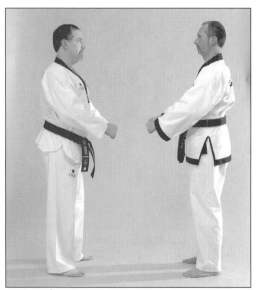

a. *Joombi* position.

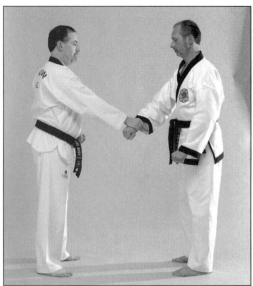

b. Attacker grabs defender's right wrist with his right hand.

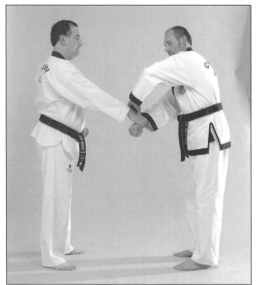

c. Reaching over, grab attacker's right hand with your left placing thumb on middle knuckle.

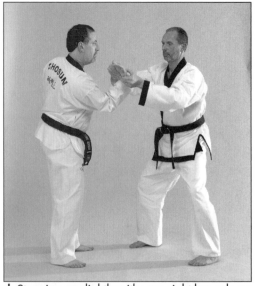

d. Stepping up slightly with your right leg, release right hand matching thumbs, then twist attacker's wrist so that the palm is facing the ground while keeping arm crooked.

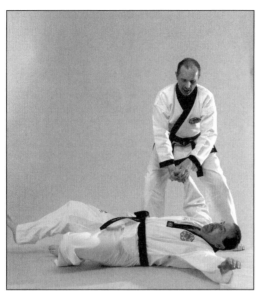

e. Stepping back with your left leg into horse stance, force opponent to ground by pushing downward with both thumbs.

Ho Sin Sool 5

(Defense against lapel grab)

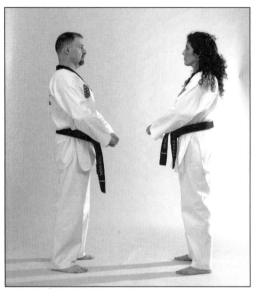

a. *Joombi* position.

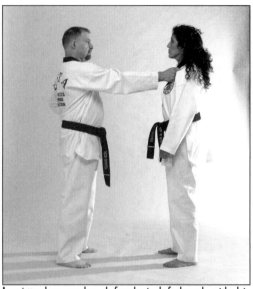

b. Attacker grabs defender's left lapel with his right hand.

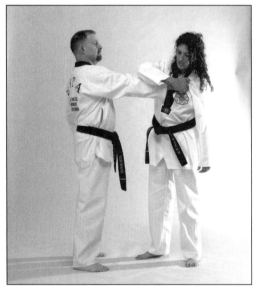

c. Turns towards attacker's right while simultaneously grabbing offending hand with your right, fingers downward.

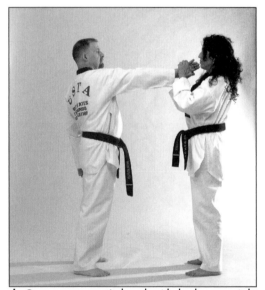

d. Grasp opponent's hand with both your right and left hands while twisting to your right.

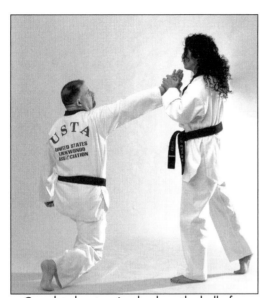

e. Complete by stepping back on the ball of your right foot, bearing down on attacker's wrist.

Ho Sin Sool 6

(Defense against cross hand grab)

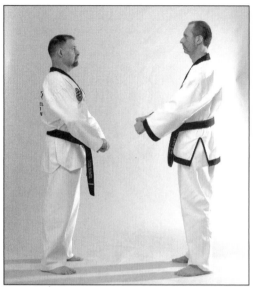

a. *Joombi* position.

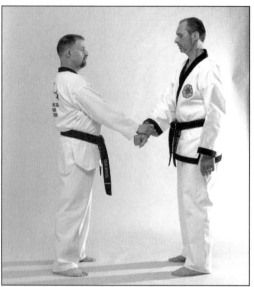

b. Attacker grabs defender's right wrist with his right hand.

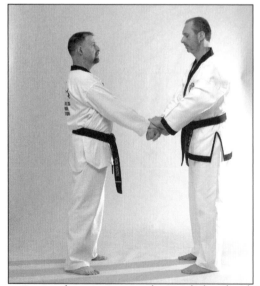

c. Capture by covering attacker's right hand with your left.

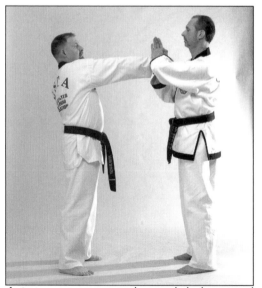

d. Swing arms in, up and around clockwise until positioned in front of chest while retaining captured hand.

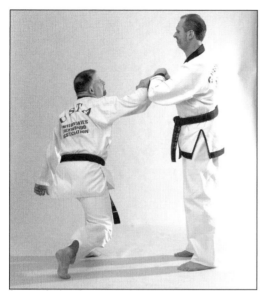

f. Finish by bearing down on attacker's right wrist.

HO SIN SOOL 7
(Defense against double hand grab from the front)

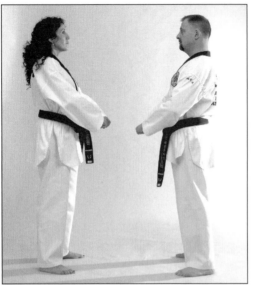

a. *Joombi* position.

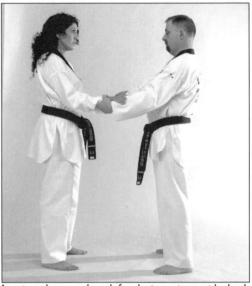

b. Attacker grabs defender's wrists with both hands.

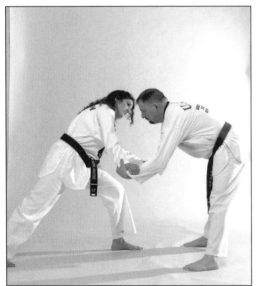

c. Defender grabs the assailant's wrists and steps back with right leg.

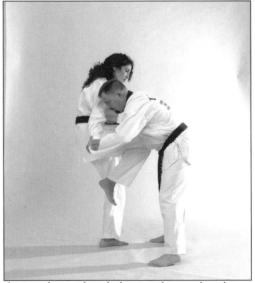

d. Complete with right knee strike to solar plexus.

HO SIN SOOL 8

(Defense against double hand grab from behind)

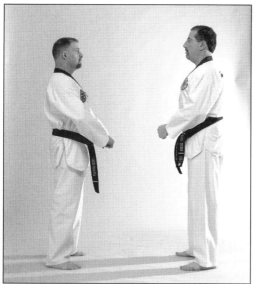

a. *Joombi* position.

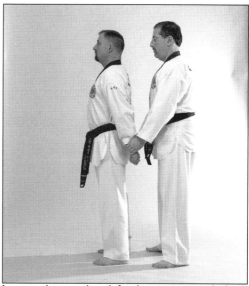

b. Attacker grabs defender's wrists with both hands from behind.

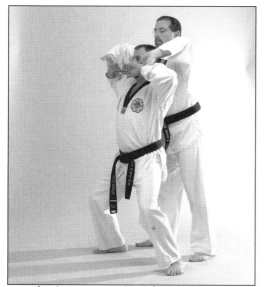

c. Defender steps to the left into horse stance while raising both elbows so that the back of the hands are at eye level.

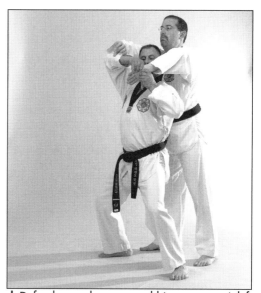

d. Defender reaches over grabbing opponent's left hand with his right while simultaneously releasing left placing both thumbs on the middle knuckle.

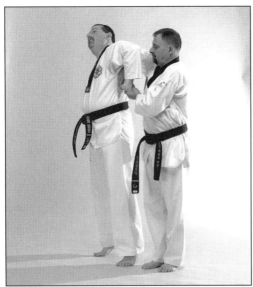

e. Step under attacker's left arm with your right shoulder, rotating wrist clockwise while keeping elbow high.

HO SIN SOOL 9

(Defense against reverse punch and lapel grab)

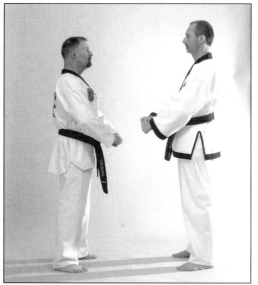

a. *Joombi* position.

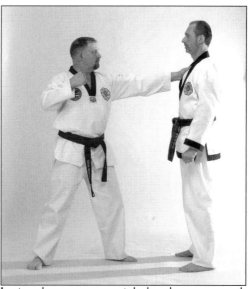

b. Attacker executes a right hand reverse punch while grabbing defender's right lapel with his left.

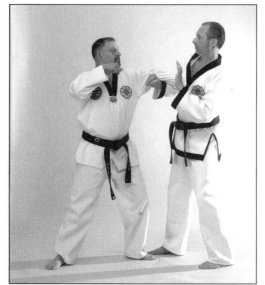

c. Defender performs a left palm heel block while simultaneously executing a right arm lock by circling the grabbing arm clockwise and placing wrist under opponent's left elbow.

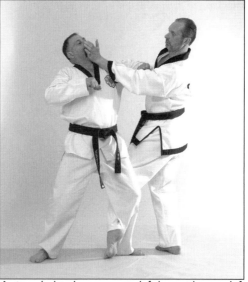

d. Step behind opponent's left leg with your left leg while executing a left hand palm heel strike to the chin, maintaining the arm lock.

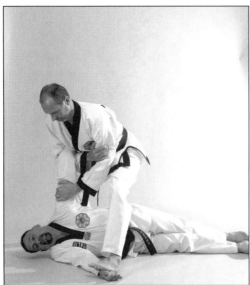

e. Sweep attacker to ground and step on his right arm to prevent a hand strike. Finish with an arm bar by grasping your upper arm with your right hand and the opponent's upper arm with your left hand, breaking the elbow.

Ho Sin Sool 10

(Defense against false handshake)

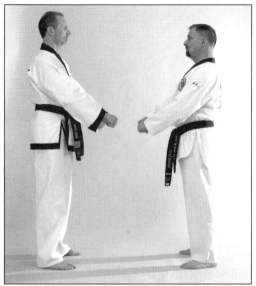

a. *Joombi* position.

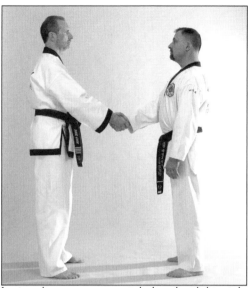

b. Attacker grasps your right hand with his right hand in a handshake.

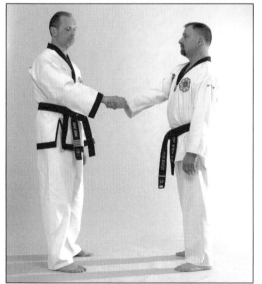

c. Defender rotates the hands counter clockwise so that his hand is on top.

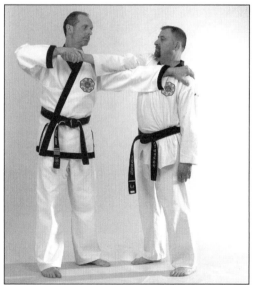

d. Thrust your left hand under the opponent's elbow and grab his left shoulder.

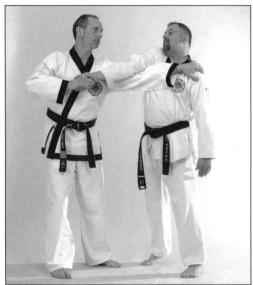

e. Complete by pressing downward, breaking the elbow on your forearm.

HO SIN SOOL 11

(Defense against side wrist grab)

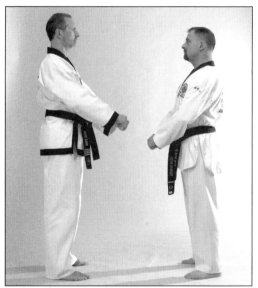

a. *Joombi* position.

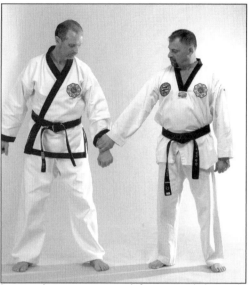

b. Attacker grasps your left wrist with his right hand, palm down.

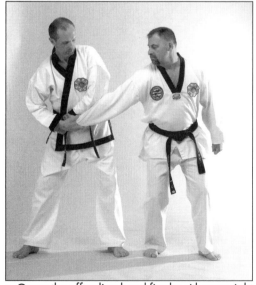

c. Grasp the offending hand firmly with your right hand while pulling straight inward and across your abdomen.

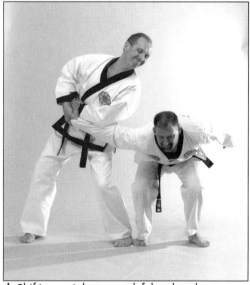

d. Shifting weight to your left leg, bend your captured arm sharply to strike downward with the point of your elbow against opponent's elbow, breaking it.

HO SIN SOOL 12

(Defense against same side grab)

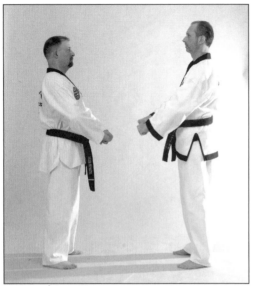

a. *Joombi* position.

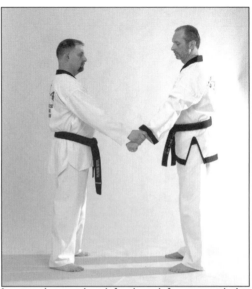

b. Attacker grabs defender's left wrist with his right hand.

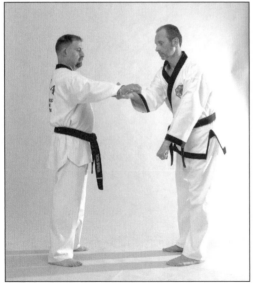

c. Defender breaks opponent's grip by slapping hand away with his right.

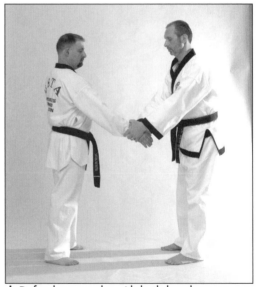

d. Defender re-grabs with both hands.

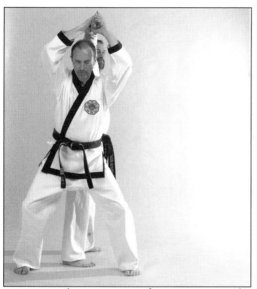

e. Assume horse stance after stepping under attacker's right arm with your right leg.

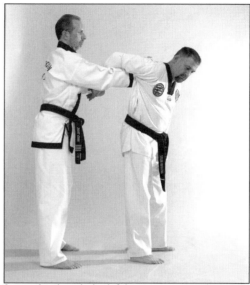

f. Step back with the left leg into an upright stance while thrusting your right arm up and under opponent's left, grabbing the back of the collar.

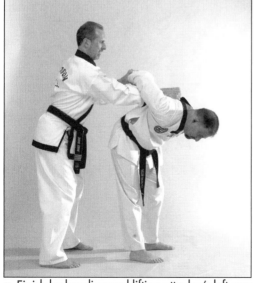

g. Finish by bending and lifting attacker's left arm with your right hand, dislocating the shoulder and breaking the elbow.

HO SIN SOOL 13
(Defense against same side grab)

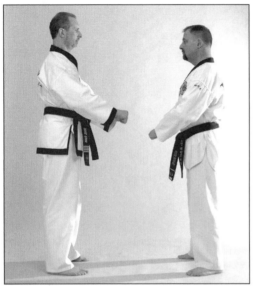

a. *Joombi* position.

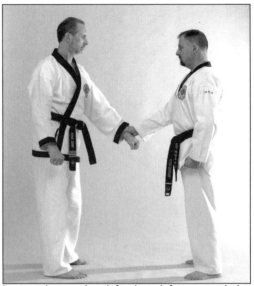

b. Attacker grabs defender's left wrist with his right hand.

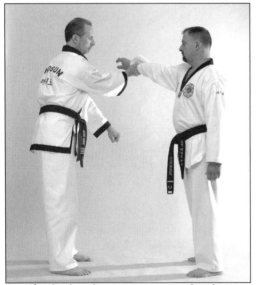

c. Defender breaks opponent's grip by slapping hand away with his right.

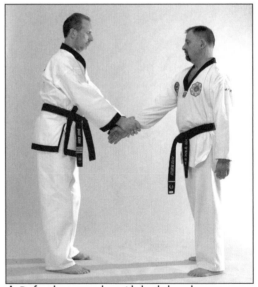

d. Defender re-grabs with both hands.

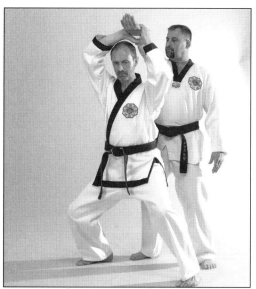

e. Assume horse stance after stepping under attacker's right arm with your left leg.

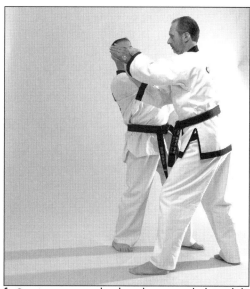

f. Continue to step back with your right leg while maintaining grip on attacker's right wrist with your left hand.

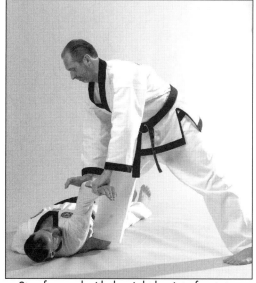

g. Step forward with the right leg into front stance while counterattacking with a right hand palm heel strike to opponent's elbow.

Ho Sin Sool 14

(Defense against downward pipe strike)

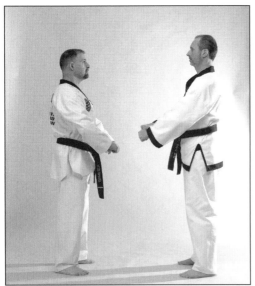

a. *Joombi* position.

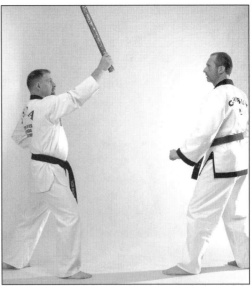

b. Attacker steps forward with his right leg while executing a downward pipe strike with the right hand.

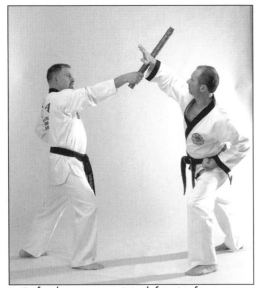

c. Defender steps up into left twist front stance while performing a right sweeping high knife hand block.

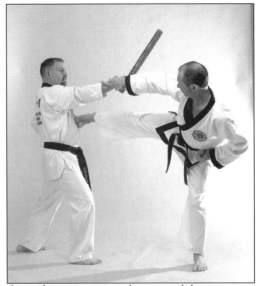

d. Grab opponent's right wrist while counterattacking with a right leg ball of foot round kick to the solar plexus.

HO SIN SOOL 15

(Defense against downward pipe strike)

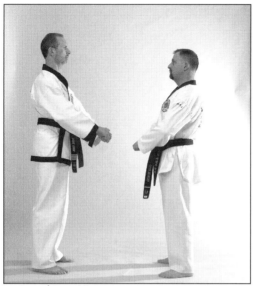

a. *Joombi* position.

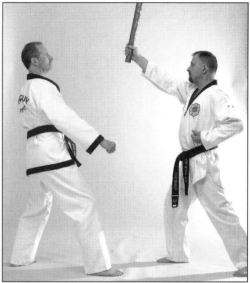

b. Attacker steps forward with his right leg while executing a downward pipe strike with the right hand.

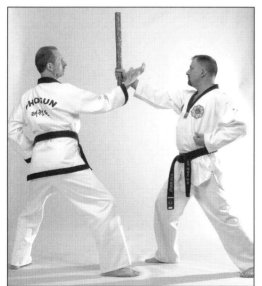

c. Defender steps back into back stance with the left leg while delivering a right out/in knife hand block.

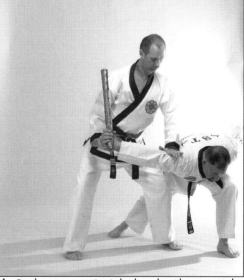

d. Grab opponent's right hand with your right, thumb on middle knuckle and step 180 degrees to your left into horse stance while executing a left palm heel strike to attacker's right shoulder joint.

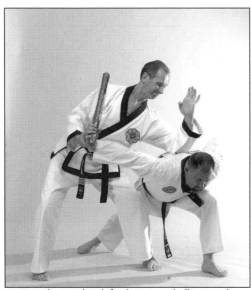

e. Complete with a left, downward elbow strike to opponent's back.

HO SIN SOOL 16

(Defense against lunging knife attack)

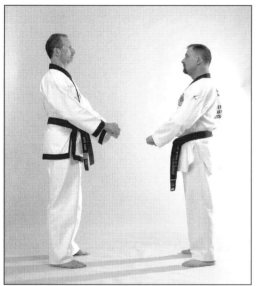

a. *Joombi* position.

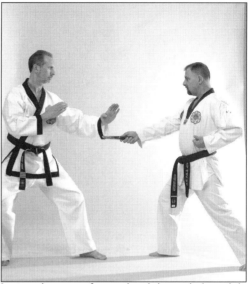

b. Attacker steps forward with his right leg while executing a lunging knife attack with the right hand.

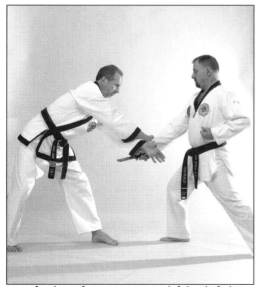

c. Defender, after assuming a left-back fighting stance, hands open, slides back one step and executes a low knife hand X block, right hand over left hand.

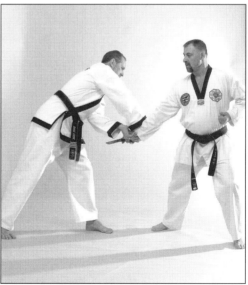

d. Rotating both hands counter clockwise, grasp the offending hand by placing both thumbs on the opponent's middle knuckle.

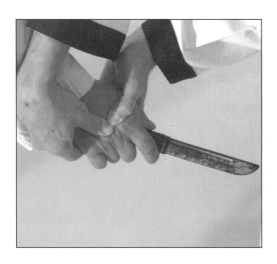

e. Close up of wrist rotation grab.

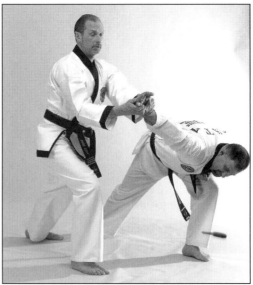

f. Step to the right into a right front stance while twisting attacker's arm up and to the right, finally forcing him to disarm by pushing the fingers towards his head.

HO SIN SOOL 17

(Defense against lunging knife attack)

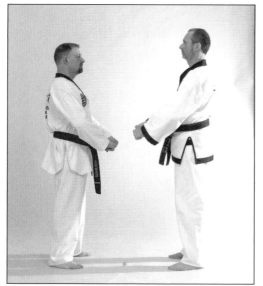

a. *Joombi* position.

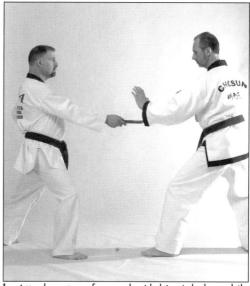

b. Attacker steps forward with his right leg while executing a lunging knife attack with the right hand.

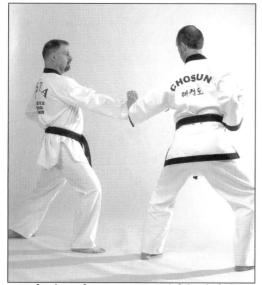

c. Defender, after assuming a left-back fighting stance, hands open, steps back 90 degrees to the right into horse stance while executing a left palm heel block to the attacker's right wrist.

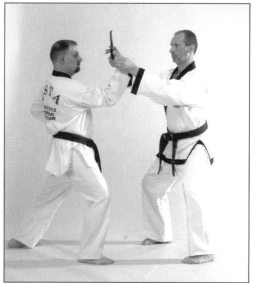

d. After grasping the offending hand with his left, thumb on the middle knuckle, the defender steps 180 degrees to the left into horse stance, grabbing with his right hand and matching thumbs.

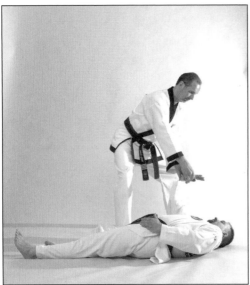

e. Stepping back with your left leg into horse stance, force the opponent to the ground by pushing downwards with both thumbs.

HO SIN SOOL 18

(Defense against downward knife attack)

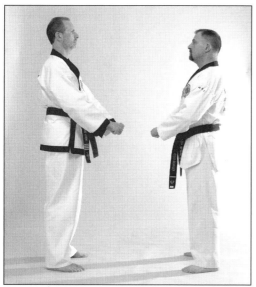

a. *Joombi* position.

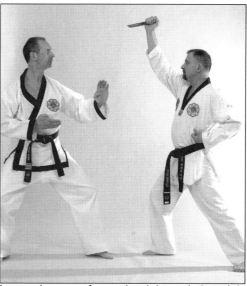

b. Attacker steps forward with his right leg while executing a downward knife attack with the right hand.

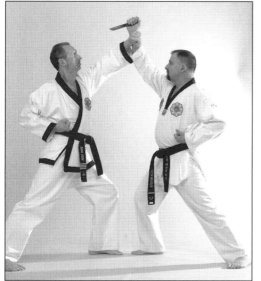

c. Defender slides his right foot back assuming a left front stance while executing a left hand high block.

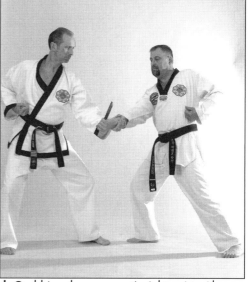

d. Grabbing the opponent's right wrist with your left hand, swing the right arm counter clockwise down and in, evading the knife.

HO SIN SOOL 18 (continued)
(Defense against downward knife attack)

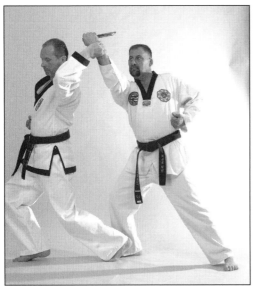

e. Continue the circle while pivoting on the balls of both feet.

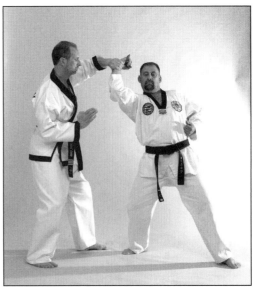

f. Slide your left foot to the left, moving your body under the opponent's offending arm.

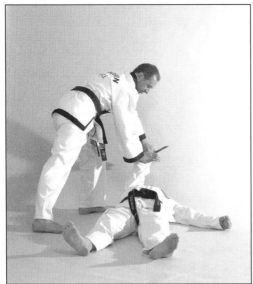

g. Step forward with your left leg while pushing forward on the attacker's elbow forcing him to ground.

CHAPTER 12
Self-Defense Practice for Women

As with any form of unarmed self-defense—speed, balance, and body mechanics, coupled with the element of surprise in tandem with a working knowledge of vital striking points—play a vital role in the ultimate success of the techniques employed. This is particularly true in the practice and application of women's self-defense tactics because females tend to be victimized by males who are stronger and outweigh them. It must be remembered that traditional taekwondo defensive strategy does not rely simply on brute force, but rather on technical proficiency and the will to, when all else fails, utilize potentially lethal skills in conjunction with the elements mentioned above.

Having said this, women practicing self-defense for the first time will invariably attempt to implement the basic skills they have learned on a loved one at home for practice. Often, one of two things will occur: either the recipient will be injured, or the technique will prove virtually ineffective. In the first case, care was not taken in the execution of the defensive measure due to inexperience, while in the second; the express will to extract oneself from an altercation through a determined response was not present. It is essential to realize that women's self-defense techniques must be applied with unparalleled commitment, presence of mind, and all the power one can muster if they are to work at all. Having no real desire to harm a boyfriend or husband in the first place will no doubt hinder the consequences of the technique being practiced possibly resulting in frustration and the false belief that the application is useless. In teaching a women's self-defense course, I constantly remind my students of the equation below:

SELF-DEFENSE SKILLS + THE WILL TO RESPOND = ESCAPE

Most women, due to the manner in which they were raised, exhibit a benign and compassionate nature in regards to self-defense. This characteristic must be overcome, if only for a moment, in the midst of a real altercation because not coupling skill with will is certain to have monumentally disastrous effects; a second chance to apply a given technique is rarely given.

Keep in mind, however, that true self-defense is not defined by the amount of injury one can inflict on an attacker, but in the ability of the potential victim to escape or evade unsullied as quickly as possible. Therefore, avoiding a threatening situation in the first place is most desirable. Avoidance techniques include:

- Steer clear of isolated areas.
- Use common sense when speaking with strangers.
- Scan your surroundings as you walk. Stay aware of your environment.
- Walk with confidence. Do not look like a victim.
- Circumvent suspicious groups of people.
- When shopping, park in lighted areas.
- Shop with a friend and not until you are exhausted.
- Return change to your wallet before leaving the cashier.
- Have your car keys out and ready to use.
- Check under your car and in the backseat before entering the vehicle.
- Avoid compromising situations with unfamiliar people.
- Do not drink from an open container at parties with unfamiliar people.
- Do not leave your drink unattended at parties.
- Do not wear expensive jewelry in strange surroundings.
- Rely on instinct; if a situation does not feel right, it probably isn't.

If you are confronted by an assailant and feel an attack is immanent, but have not yet been physically assaulted, immediately respond with one or all of the following:

- Remain calm. Breathe deeply.
- If possible, run as quickly as you can from the area.
- Do not aggravate the aggressor with violent language.
- Request assistance from a passerby.
- Make a loud noise to draw attention to yourself. Carry a whistle.
- Feign sickness.
- If your assailant wants material possessions, give them to him.

If avoiding an altercation is not possible and the use of martial arts techniques remains the only option, then as with avoidance, there a several key factors to remember:

- Try not to panic. Maintain presence of mind. Breathe deeply.
- Use the element of surprise to your advantage.
- Choose your target carefully before you strike.
- Execute the chosen techniques with total commitment.

While the techniques described below are simple and fast to execute, they are by no means exclusive to women's self-defense. Rather, they are universal traditional taekwondo skills. They have been chosen for this book however, for their simplicity and ease of use; two crucial elements of practical self-defense. During the initial practice of these traditional taekwondo defensive strategies a number of cautionary measures should be followed:

- Always use caution during practice.
- Do not develop a "false sense of security."
- Practice slowly and deliberately in the beginning.
- Approach the application of these techniques with utmost seriousness as though you were truly being attacked.
- These techniques must become ingrained if they are to be effective.

Finally, it is wise to use a technique to the point of submission, then escape. Remember: the ultimate goal of self-defense is to escape unharmed, not simply to injure your attacker.

WOMEN'S SELF-DEFENSE DRILLS—WOMEN'S SELF-DEFENSE TECHNIQUE 1: THE FIST
Primary Striking Areas: Face, Solar Plexus.

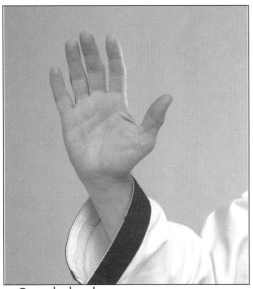

a. Open the hand.

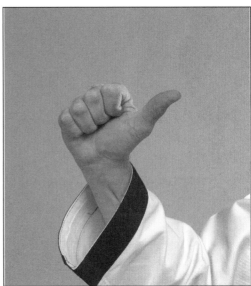

b. Clinch the fingers tightly against the palm.

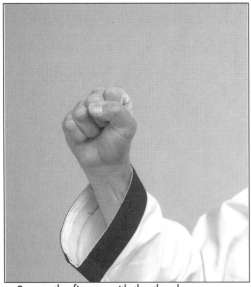

c. Secure the fingers with the thumb.

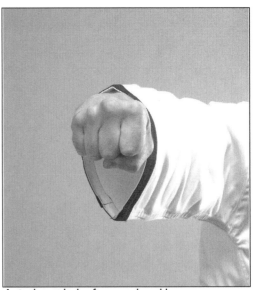

d. Strike with the first two knuckles.

WOMEN'S SELF-DEFENSE TECHNIQUE 2: THE DEFENSE STANCE

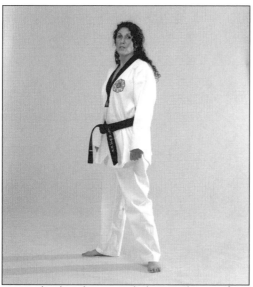

a. Step back with your right leg 45 degrees from center, legs shoulder width apart maintaining height advantage.

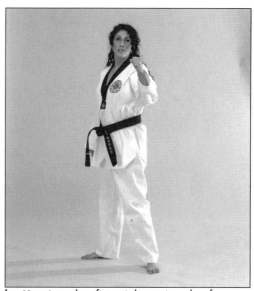

b. Keeping the fists tight, raise the front or "guard" hand to protect your face and head.

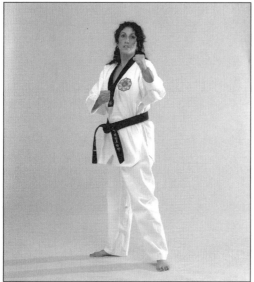

c. Position the rear hand and arm in preparation for a strike and to protect your rib area.

WOMEN'S SELF-DEFENSE TECHNIQUE 3: THE KIHOP

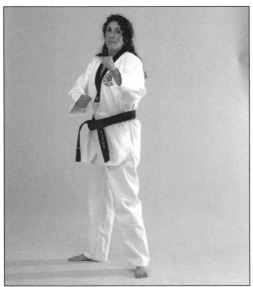

a. Breathe in deeply.

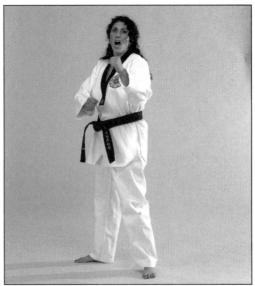

b. Emit a yell from the solar plexus meant to startle your assailant. The yell should annunciate the sound *"kihop!"*

WOMEN'S SELF-DEFENSE TECHNIQUE 4: THE JAB/REVERSE PUNCH COMBINATION

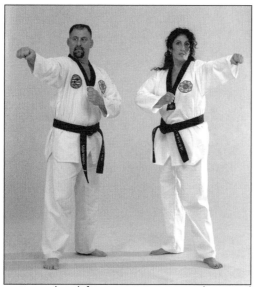 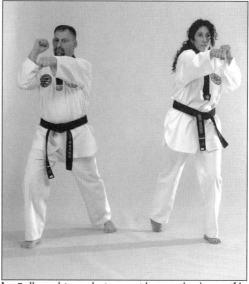

a. From the defense stance, project the guard hand forward striking with the first two knuckles.

b. Follow this technique with a strike by swiftly extending the rear hand, also using the first two knuckles.

WOMEN'S SELF-DEFENSE TECHNIQUE 5: THE BACK FIST
Primary Striking Areas: Bridge of the Nose, Jaw, Temple, Ear, Eye.

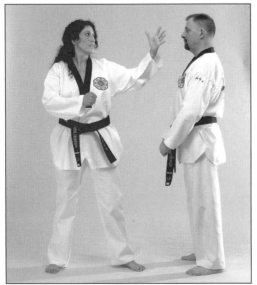

a. Open the fingers of the guard hand.

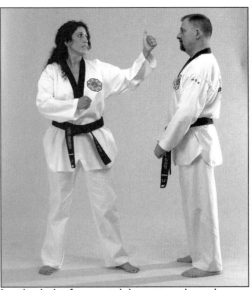

b. Clinch the fingers tightly against the palm.

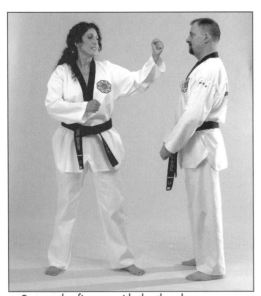

c. Secure the fingers with the thumb.

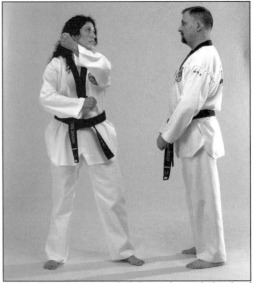

d. Bending the wrist slightly, strike with back of the first two knuckles.

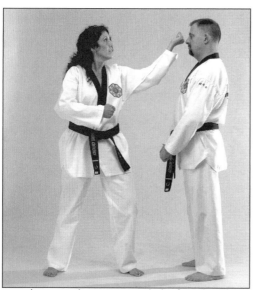 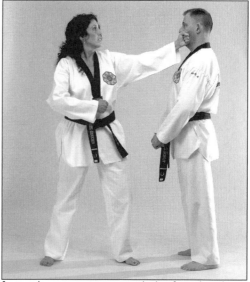

e. A downward trajectory with the front hand can be used.

f. A sideways trajectory with the front hand can be used.

WOMEN'S SELF-DEFENSE TECHNIQUE 6: THE PALM HEEL STRIKE
Primary Striking Areas: Solar Plexus, Chin, Nose.

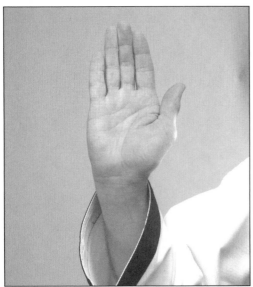 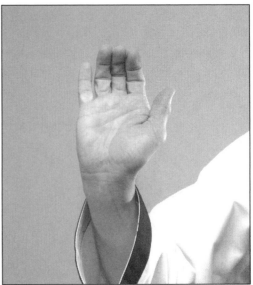

a. Hold the hand open and bent slightly at the wrist.

b. The fingers and thumb are curved and held away from the palm.

WOMEN'S SELF-DEFENSE TECHNIQUE 7: FIVE ELBOW STRIKES

Primary Striking Areas: Chin, Back, Jaw, Temple and Ribs, Solar Plexus, and Groin (used primarily for close-quarters defense).

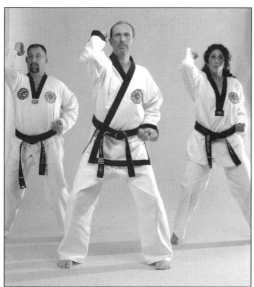

a. Upward elbow strike.

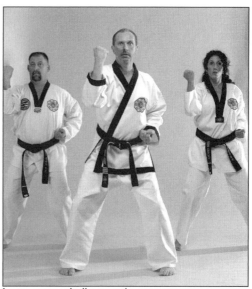

b. Downward elbow strike.

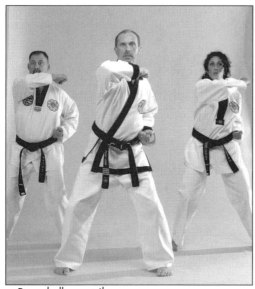

c. Round elbow strike.

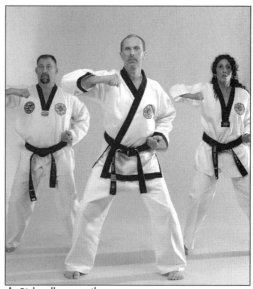

d. Side elbow strike.

WOMEN'S SELF-DEFENSE TECHNIQUE 7: FIVE ELBOW STRIKES (CONTINUED)

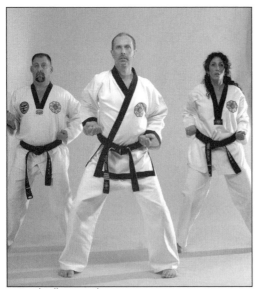

e. Back elbow strike.

WOMEN'S SELF-DEFENSE TECHNIQUE 8: KNEE STRIKE

Primary Striking Areas: Groin, Solar Plexus, Face (often used in conjunction with a shoulder grab).

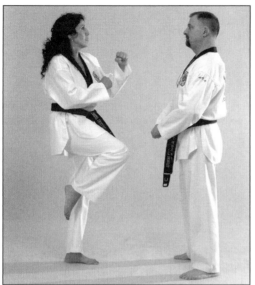 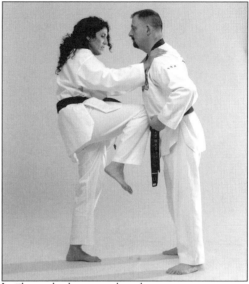

a. From a defense stance, bend the leg.

b. Thrust the knee up sharply.

WOMEN'S SELF-DEFENSE TECHNIQUE 9: FRONT KICK

Primary Striking Areas: Groin (instep), Solar Plexus, Face (ball of foot).

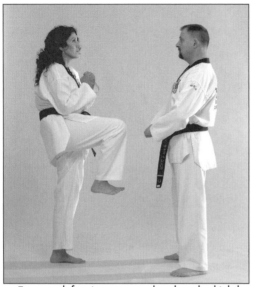

a. From a defensive stance, chamber the kick by bending the leg at the knee.

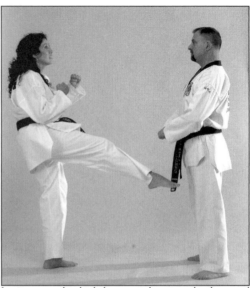

b. Execute the kick by straightening the leg and striking with either the instep or the ball of the foot.

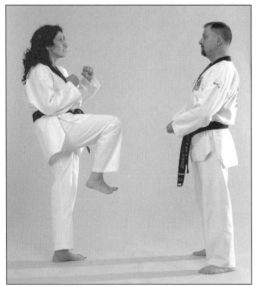

c. Retract the leg at he knee to avoid being grabbed.

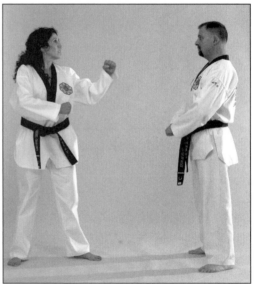

d. Step back into a defensive stance.

WOMEN'S SELF-DEFENSE TECHNIQUE 10: FRONT LEG ROUND KICK
Primary Striking Areas: Stomach, Face, Back of Thigh.

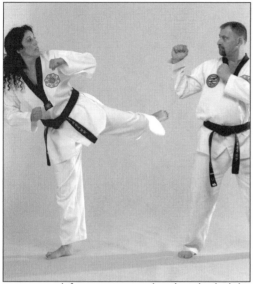

a. From a defensive stance, chamber the kick by lifting the front leg and bending the knee, heel to the buttocks.

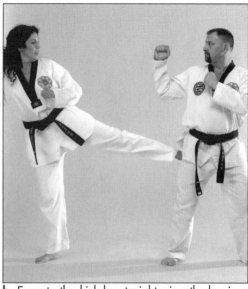

b. Execute the kick by straightening the leg in a trajectory parallel to the floor, striking with the instep.

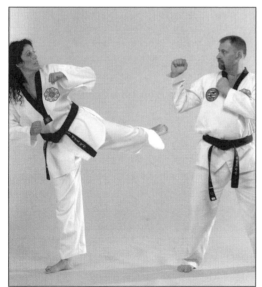

c. Retract the leg at he knee to avoid being grabbed.

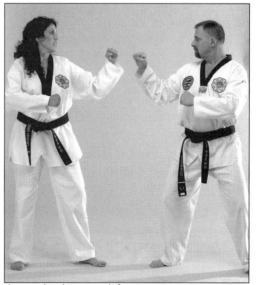

d. Step back into a defensive stance.

WOMEN'S SELF-DEFENSE TECHNIQUE 11: DEFENSE AGAINST CHOKE

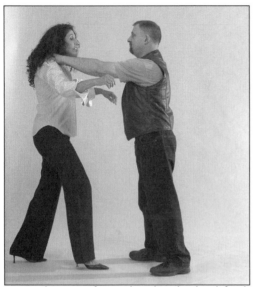 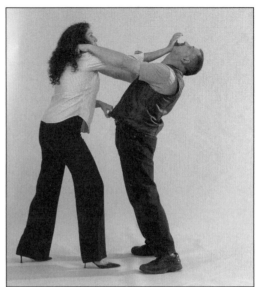

a. Attacker steps forward and grabs the defender with both hands around the neck.

b. Defender pulls of the opponent's belt or pants front while simultaneously executing a palm heel strike to the chin.

WOMEN'S SELF-DEFENSE TECHNIQUE 12: DEFENSE AGAINST DOUBLE LAPEL GRAB

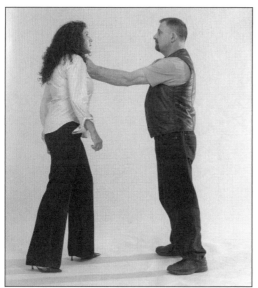

a. Attacker steps forward and grabs the defender by the lapels or the front of the blouse with both hands.

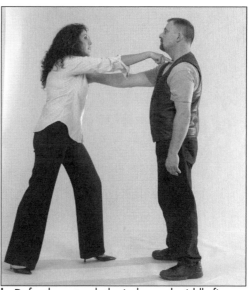

b. Defender extends the index and middle fingers straight out and pushes sharply in on the soft portion of the opponent's throat.

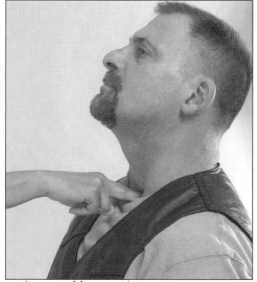

c. Close up of finger strike.

WOMEN'S SELF-DEFENSE TECHNIQUE 13: DEFENSE AGAINST BEAR HUG FROM BEHIND

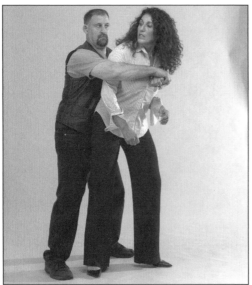

a. Attacker performs a bear hug to the defender from behind.

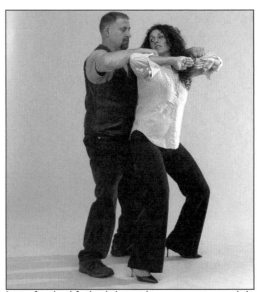

b. Defender lifts both legs, dropping center, while raising both elbows so that the back of the hands are at eye level, loosening opponent's grip.

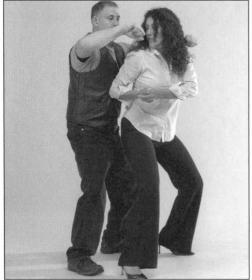

c. Finish with a back elbow strike to attacker's groin or solar plexus.

WOMEN'S SELF-DEFENSE TECHNIQUE 14: DEFENSE AGAINST CHEST GRAB

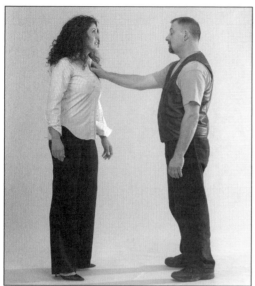

a. Attacker grabs defender's chest with his right hand.

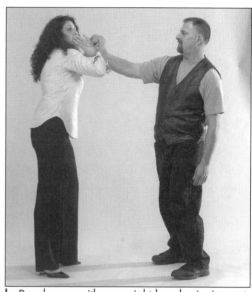

b. Reach over with your right hand gripping outside of attacker's hand while placing thumb on middle knuckle.

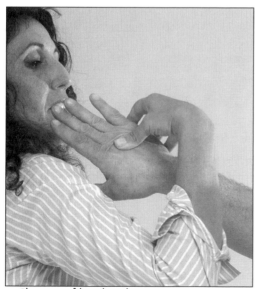

c. Close up of hand grab

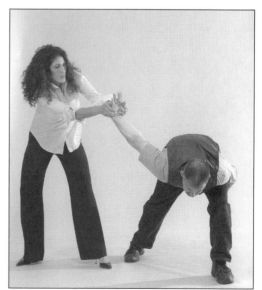

d. Continue by grabbing opponent's hand with your left, matching thumbs, and twisting clockwise until the attacker's fingers are pointing upward.

WOMEN'S SELF-DEFENSE TECHNIQUE 14: DEFENSE AGAINST CHEST GRAB
(CONTINUED)

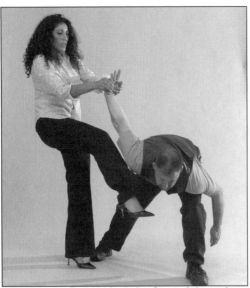

e. Execute a front kick to the face while pushing fingers towards the opponent's head.

WOMEN'S SELF-DEFENSE TECHNIQUE 15: DEFENSE AGAINST THROAT/ARM HOLD FROM BEHIND

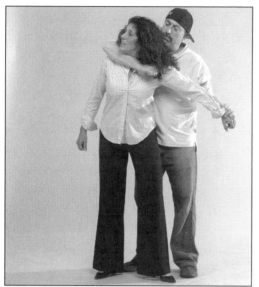

a. Attacker grabs defender around the neck with his right arm, while holding the left wrist with his left.

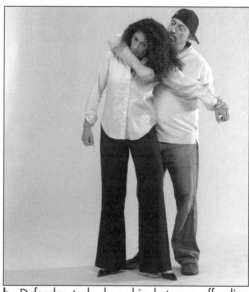

b. Defender tucks her chin between offending arm and the throat to allow the passage of air.

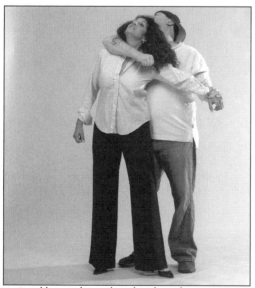

c. Quickly employ a head to butt the opponent's face.

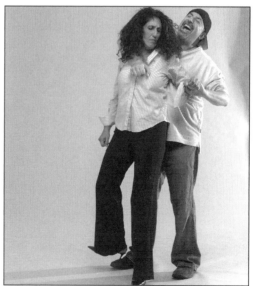

d. Scraping the attacker's shin with the right foot, stomp down on the instep.

WOMEN'S SELF-DEFENSE TECHNIQUE 15: DEFENSE AGAINST THROAT/ARM HOLD FROM BEHIND
(CONTINUED)

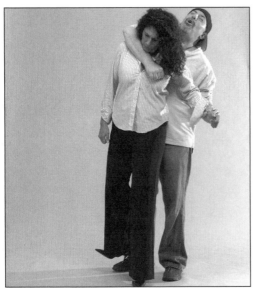

e. Finish by executing a back elbow strike to the solar plexus.

Women's Self-Defense Technique 16: Defense Against Bear Hug From The Front

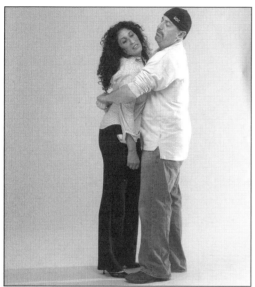

a. Attacker performs a bear hug to the defender from the front.

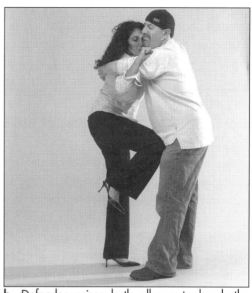

b. Defender raises both elbows to break the attacker's hold while simultaneously executing a knee strike to the groin.

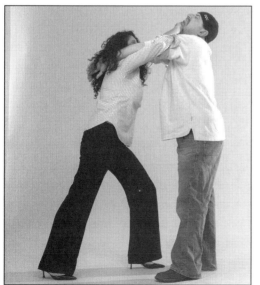

c. Reach up and over opponent's arms placing the left palm on the chin and the right palm on the back of your left hand.

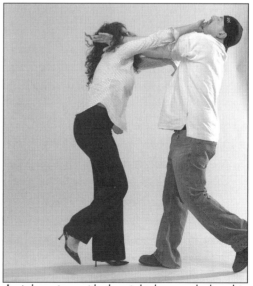

d. Advancing with the right leg, push the chin with a strong forward motion.

Conclusion

Although traditional taekwondo is highly democratic in nature, attracting a diverse cross-section of the population, it nevertheless requires a strong character coupled with a genuine desire to succeed. By way of example, one must prioritize their time in order to attend classes on a consistent basis irrespective of a hectic schedule, and in the course of achieving measurable goals not be overly swayed by the specter of self-criticism. Since the very foundation of the martial arts rests on philosophical paradigms intrinsically foreign to the Western mind, the novice must empty the cup of preconceived notions and be willing to accept metaphysical and cultural concepts that are often contradictory to those they have become familiar with since childhood. The physical body, too, is routinely put to the test by being asked to perform exercises that, in all likelihood, have never been attempted before. These hurdles quickly lead to the realization that the practice of traditional taekwondo is not for everyone; if it were easy, if there existed and elevator to the top floor of proficiency, schools around the globe would be filled to capacity with eager, but apathetic students largely driven by the cinematic engine that glorifies empty-hand combat.

Yet, there are those who do not seek to emulate the martial arts stars of stage and screen, choosing instead to fulfill an innate desire to fortify their mind, body, and spirit through the ritualized practice of an authentic, traditional martial art. Not feeling the need to fly through the air, vanquish armies of attackers, or don gaudy fighting attire, it is they who will persevere through the days and years of difficult training while nurturing a noble heart. Undoubtedly seeking the quiet confidence and resolve of the true martial artist, the man, woman, or child who steps across the threshold of the training hall for the first time will not be the same person on the occasion when the black belt is fitted around their waist by a master instructor. They will have developed, by then, attributes that only a sincere practice of traditional taekwondo can afford—grace will be enhanced through economy of motion; an increase in stamina due to vigorous physical exercise will quickly become apparent; improved focus and concentration will result from repeated sessions of meditation and *Ki* development exercises. In addition to a multitude of other virtues, a general sense of well being will by then be realized linked to an appreciation for one's unique place in the universe.

Looking back over the formative years of the Korean martial arts, we have seen that the double-edged sword of courage and nobility successfully cut a path for the unification of the Three Kingdoms. Because traditional taekwondo traces its heritage to the actions of the Hwarang and Hwarang-do, the philosophical doctrine that strategically advocated dignity and honor in battle, we can therefore conclude that the national martial art of Korea is not only an effective means of self-defense and self-enrichment as stated above, but a moral compass pointing the way to nobility as well. Certainly, nobility supported by courage exists today in the hearts and minds of many individuals young and old alike but needs to be drawn out and nurtured. Since the root of the word education can be construed as the process of drawing out, then martial arts training can be used as a vehicle for this purpose by those predisposed to its virtues. Certainly, the techniques illustrated in this book and others of similar design, will appear difficult to the faint of heart, yet not to those who have cultivated patience and determination, courage and compassion through traditional taekwondo training. These characteristics identify a martial artist in the truest sense of the word and act as a bridge between the physical component of taekwondo training and an enlightened way of life. Gazing out over a group of meditating students in repose, an experienced instructor can sense the collective nobility of those assembled as it permeates the *dojang*. These are no ordinary people; most dedicated practitioners devote many hours a week to their training in harmony with work, school, and household responsibilities. The rewards, however, are clear in that life, with its pitfalls and its pleasures, is appreciated in its fullness as a direct result of diligent training coupled with the Zen practice of living in the moment; a highly difficult state of mind to achieve yet an essential element of traditional taekwondo.

Naturally, the only sure method of navigating the summit to enlightenment through the martial arts is to take the high road as it relates to the traditional taekwondo curriculum and the comprehensive training program it offers. Nobility, virtue, and effective technique cannot prosper unless it is fed an ample diet of holistic training; *poom-se* will suffer at the hands of poor basic technique. Self-defense practice will collapse under the weight of a feeble will left exposed by an ignorance of *Ki*. The intensity and tempo of a taekwondo class is certain to overwhelm those lacking the indomitable spirit required to push their body to its limits. A wise instructor must therefore foster ability while running the risk of creating an ingredient of stress in his students by demanding more of the individual then they think themselves capable of physically, mentally, and spiritually—something that happens rarely in the modern school environment where dollars often triumph over tradition. Any worthwhile pursuit clearly presents a challenge; the magnitude of that challenge is a function of the expectations the participants superimpose on themselves. From white belt to black belt and beyond, these expectations appear to compound at a dizzying rate. Yet it is a sincere love for the martial arts supported by the motivation of a competent instructor that continues to drive the practitioner to new heights of proficiency.

Traditional taekwondo, complete with its physical, spiritual, and academic components, represents a body of knowledge that is extremely fulfilling yet, as we have come to see, demanding of time, energy, and focus. Nevertheless, it is a fact that those rising to the challenge, those with the patience and fortitude to forge a clear path through adversity, complacency, and the hundreds of excuses one can conjure up on any one given day to avoid training, will, instead of coming to taekwondo, become taekwondo.

Train hard, remain focused, and in the words of Grandmaster Richard Chun: "Never give up!"

Master Doug Cook
September 2005

APPENDIX A

Training in Korea with Grandmaster Gyoo Hyun Lee

At one time or another, almost every martial artist dreams of visiting the country from which their chosen discipline has evolved. To the *karateka*, that region is Japan; to the *gungfu* practitioner, it is China. However, to the taekwondoist, it is a peninsula rich in greenery, the size of Indiana, with mountains masked in swirling mists that rush to meet the sky. This enchanted nation is called Korea: Land of the Morning Calm. Couple this desire with the opportunity to train alongside a revered icon in the martial arts community and you are presented with a winning formula for a highly rewarding excursion.

Paging through the *Kukkiwon Textbook* many years ago, I took notice of a severe looking martial artist chosen to model the unique and effective techniques of taekwondo by virtue of his long experience and skilled attention to detail. Again, in 1998, this high-ranking practitioner would appear to me as a staff instructor in a promotional video for the Organizing Committee for Taekwondo Korea 2000. Seeing Grandmaster Gyoo Hyun Lee in action rather than on the printed page, convinced me beyond the shadow of a doubt that someday I would seek out his instruction. As destiny would have it, this was more difficult than expected.

In planning the 1999 United States Taekwondo Association Korea Training & Cultural Tour, I had inquired if Grandmaster Lee would be one of our teachers and was informed that his schedule did not coincide with our visit. Subsequently, in the initial planning stage of the 2004 Chosun Taekwondo Academy Training & Cultural Tour, I once more requested his talents. "Unavailable", was the response from Korea and so, disappointedly, I turned my gaze elsewhere. Then, a few short weeks before our departure in June 2004, I received a surprise email from our travel agent in Seoul, stating that the grandmaster had accepted our group for a day of training provided we allow his senior instructors to assist. This stipulation took all of one minute to consider. Rather than a condition, it was truly a bonus!

Following breakfast on our fourth day of training in Korea, we boarded a motor coach and began the journey to Yangsu-ri, a small village about an hour's drive from

Seoul. Our training to date at Kyung Won University and HOKI Taekwondo had been challenging and highly rewarding, balanced between the martial art and combat sport of taekwondo. Today's training, however, would focus on precise basic technique and the pursuit of excellence in *poom-se,* the formal exercises unique to taekwondo.

The metropolitan scenery flashed by as our guide directed us to turn our attention to several key points of interest along the way. Slowly, the urban sprawl began to thin as rice fields replaced the high-rise apartments. We exited the freeway and snaked our way through winding country roads barely wide enough to accommodate the width of our bus. A tiny picturesque village materialized with a gas station, restaurant, and shops selling fish, red peppers and an assortment of daily needs.

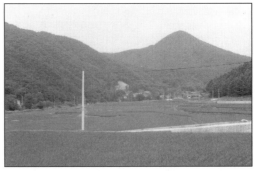

Rice fields below the dojang.

Crossing a well-maintained concrete bridge minus guard rails that spanned a swiftly running brook, we had gone as far as our bus could take us. As the doors opened, I was the second person off after our driver who was animatedly chatting with two gentlemen standing next to a Hyundai sedan. I was suddenly overwhelmed with awe as I saw the grandmaster we had traveled eight thousand miles to train with before me. Single file, my students lined up and bowed. It was then that the stern face I had only witnessed in photos and on film erupted into a broad, welcoming smile. Grandmaster Lee invited us to follow him and his instructors up a rutted dirt road.

We passed a squat, single-story dwelling on our left that is his home, and then continued on a few steps to a red brick building with two sets of double doors thrown

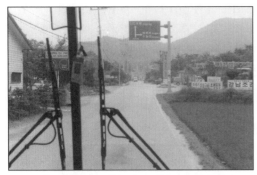

The Village of Yangsu-ri through the windscreen of our motorcoach.

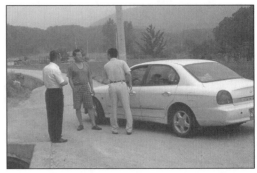

Grandmaster Lee awaiting our arrival.

open to the outside that housed the grand-master's personal dojang. Inside, it was cool in stark contrast to the humid air that weighed heavy in the small valley. Instantly, we were enchanted by our sur-roundings. The floor was set with green puzzle-mat bordered in orange, and the walls were adorned with memorabilia from a lifetime devoted to the Korean martial arts. In a neat row, over the doors, hung cir-cular metal plates inscribed with the names

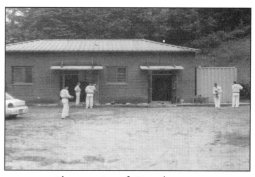

The exterior of Grandmaster Gyoo Hyun-Lee's dojang.

of the original *kwans*, or martial arts schools, established in the 1940s and 1950s, before the discordant styles were united to form taekwondo. There, names like the Moo Duk Kwan, Chung Do Kwan, and Oh Do Kwan leap out reminding us of the tenure and seniority Grandmaster Lee enjoys in the taekwondo community.

Suspended on the far wall in a black wooden frame hung a scroll written in *hangul* characters reading: "A National Sport, Taekwondo." Fifty of these icons

were said to be painted in the personal calligraphy of the late South Korean President Chung Hee Park in March of 1971. The majority, such as the one that was displayed before us, reside inside the borders of Korea while the remaining few were distributed to master instructors throughout the world. One was exhibited in Grandmaster Richard Chun's New York City *dojang* for over thirty years and was recently presented to our school as a treasured gift.

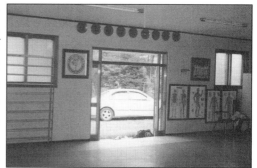

Brass plates bearing the names of the original kwans.

With reverence, we quietly prepared to train by changing into our *doboks* and lin-ing up, four across. Finally, there before us was the man the World Taekwondo Federation has endorsed as the standard against which all practitioners of taekwondo should be compared for excellence in basic motions and *poom-se*. Only recently it was brought to my attention that Grandmaster Lee and his colleague, Master Kook Hyun Jung, were chosen by the WTF to model in a series of instructional DVDs aimed at standardizing the *Taegeuk*, *Palgwe* and WTF-series black belt series *poom-se*. These DVDs, presented by Dartfish of Korea will be used as a reference tool in training referees, coaches, instructors and competitors to participate in the 2006 WTF Poom-Se World Championships in Seoul, South Korea.

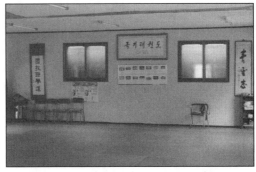

The interior of Grandmaster Lee's dojang with taekwondo scroll proudly displayed.

Both in the media and in person, Grandmaster Gyoo Hyun Lee cuts a striking image; with a shock of white hair centered over the left eye, in concert with his drill sergeant demeanor, his presence is unmistakable. Although in his early sixties, he moves like a cat. His flexibility, enthusiasm, and strength are in direct proportion to his long years of dedication to the art of taekwondo. He is currently president of the World Taekwondo Instructor Academy and director of the Kukkiwon Taekwondo Training Center. From 1990 to 1998, his abilities earned him the position of Chairman of the Training Subcommittee, Kukkiwon, and prior to that, from 1973 to 1982, he was head of the Kukkiwon Demonstration Team. Knowing this, I respectfully approached him and offered up a letter of greeting drafted by Grandmaster Chun introducing me as one of his senior students and briefly describing my qualifications. He accepted it with the humility one would expect from a man contented and secure with his place in the universe. Returning to my position in line, we assumed the joombi posture, bowed, and the training session officially began.

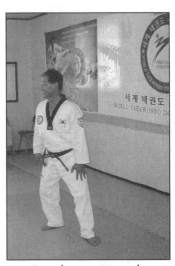

Grandmaster Lee at the head of the class.

The tension our group was projecting immediately shattered as the grandmaster, smiling, began to wiggle from side to side, shaking his arms up and down in an effort meant to relax our taut bodies. Then, reminded to breathe, the standard warm-up and flexibility exercises began in earnest. It appeared many of the more extreme postures had been borrowed from yoga. We began to perspire as the heat from our bodies warmed the room. We continued by working on technique that many would accuse of being far too simple in exchange for an eight-thousand mile trip.

My students and I, however, were so intrigued when the grandmaster reviewed the process of making a proper fist that we photographed the precision with which it was accomplished along with the wear and tear that is a result of striking solid objects for many years. Happily, our training did not stop there; front stance, back stance, middle blocks, knife hand blocks, front kicks, round kicks, and side kicks were all scrutinized beneath the magnifying glass of experience. A common thread running through the execution of every strike or block was the constant reminder

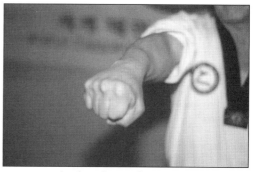

The fist of Grandmaster Lee.

to relax in our delivery and tense at the point of impact and penetration of the target. The phrase, "relaxation and POWER!" was repeated over and over again by the instructors present.

After several hours of uninterrupted training, a break was called and we congregated in small groups to compare notes and review what had been demonstrated. Some gravitated to the water cooler situated in a corner of the room for a sip of much-needed refreshment. The conversation turned to differences some were noticing in the fabric of instruction. However, before I could gain a better understanding concerning the root of these questions, we were commanded to reconvene.

At the close of the opening ritual, we were separated into groups according to belt rank and prepared for *poom-se* practice. Clearly, for black belts and color belts alike, no banquet was ever as bountiful as that day's forms practice; each was afforded the opportunity to refine the basic skills contained within the *poom-se* unique to their belt level. They were either under the intense scrutiny of Grandmaster Lee, or one of his accomplished instructors. I was working on *poom-se Pyongwon* and *Sipjin* while other black belts were focusing on *Keumgang* and *Koryo*.

I could still not believe that I was receiving private instruction from Grandmaster Gyoo Hyun Lee who patiently explained the practical application of each movement of my form in conjunction with its proper trajectory and chamber. From the corner of my eye, I glimpsed my students receiving equal attention in analyzing the various *Taegeuk poom-se* albeit with some minor alterations from what they had become accustomed

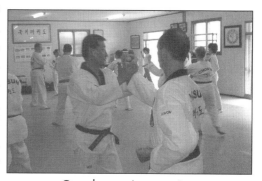

Grandmaster Lee examines
Master Doug Cook's middle block.

to. Although the *Palgwe* set was not given much credence, the eight *Taegeuk*, in tandem with the mandatory WTF black belt series *poom-se*, were thankfully addressed in detail. One refinement that I found of interest was the first preparatory motion in *poom-se Koryo* consisting of a pushing block, or *momtang milgi makki*. Having performed this form both in class and in competition on countless occasions, I had become use to projecting my hands forward with palms facing outward, thumbs a fraction of an inch apart, describing a triangle of sorts. Instead, Grandmaster Lee directed us to extend the hands forward as before, but with the palms turned inward and the thumbs slightly hooked similarly to where they would be placed when executing a knife hand technique, or *sonnal*. Although the practical application of this block is to intercept an incoming head butt, it has several less obvious functions as well. In his most recent book, *Taekwondo: Spirit and Practice*, Grandmaster Richard Chun states that this technique, which he refers to as "barrel pushing block," is a physical expression of firmness and resoluteness, demonstrating the confidence and strong will of the Korean people.

Another surprising variance came in the form of the footwork used in front stance, or ap koobi, when stepping forward in conjunction with a variety of blocks and strikes. Rather than the C-step that is commonly taught in WTF-style taekwondo, the instructors of the World Taekwondo Instructor Academy suggested we move in a more linear fashion vaguely reminiscent of the wave motion subscribed to by practitioners of the International Taekwon-Do Federation (ITF). When teaching the dynamics of the out-to-in middle block, or *ahn momtang makki*, Grandmaster Lee truly personified the essence of grace which can be defined as economy of motion. Manipulating our wrists with hands inculcated with knowledge, he described the proper height and fist rotation that added to the efficiency of the technique.

Suddenly, as the day progressed a potential dilemma began to gnaw at me, as it must many instructors from time to time, and I sensed what it was my students were referring to earlier as "differences" in curriculum. The World Taekwondo Instructor Academy under the direction of Grandmaster Gyoo Hyun Lee, is attempting, at least on the surface, to introduce a subtle shift in the dynamic principles of taekwondo technique based on an advanced understanding of physics as it relates to body mechanics. A modern approach, authored by Grandmaster Lee, is being applied to footwork, power ratio, chambering and weapons training while all the while attempting to maintain the value of traditionalism. That day in a small village on the outskirts of Seoul, we were exposed to technical variations that faintly contradict the manner of execution we had become familiar with, forcing my students to ask politely, "What do we do now?" Buried in this question is an important lesson both for my colleagues and me. Traditional taekwondo is a cultural treasure chest filled with effective self-defense skills supported by a virtuous philosophy. Although the Korean discipline contains immutable tools such as the round kick, back fist, and knife block to name a few, the manner in which these are performed may vary slightly from master to master. This fact does not corrupt the basic principles of taekwondo; rather it adds color and individuality to something that is an art rather an absolute science. Consequently, it is my desire to expose my students, at least those capable of sustaining an open mind, to the diversity inherent in taekwondo whether it is at home or abroad, resulting in what I hope will be perceived as an enhanced training experience overall. Having said this, however, it is to the teachings of my instructor, Grandmaster Richard Chun, that I am faithful.

Finally, in comparison to prior visits to Korea, the homeland of taekwondo, I could not have been more delighted in the direction our training had taken during this excursion. Thinking back, in candid discussions with several Korean practitioners during a trip in 1999, I was told of a movement initiated by local masters to return from a strictly sports-oriented approach to a more holistic style of training including forms and self-defense drills. Our experiences that day at Grandmaster Lee's *dojang*, and the days previous at Kyung Won University and HOKI Taekwondo seemed to confirm the reality of this trend. Nevertheless, to illuminate every nuance of our training under Grandmaster Gyoo Hyun Lee within the spotlight of specificity would require a great deal of editorial space and patience on the part of the reader. Therefore, it is my intention to underscore only the highlights of our experiences with this highly capable international master instructor. I am certain that future articles by other authors will be spawned in the hope of conveying the detail and value of these and other incredible training opportunities to our readers. Furthermore, it would be wise for instructors and students alike to obtain the comprehensive DVD set featuring Grandmaster Lee and sanctioned by the World Taekwondo Federation, in an effort to standardize the *Taegeuk*, *Palgwe*, and WTF-series black belt forms worldwide.

Master Doug Cook, a 4th Dan black belt, is head instructor of the Chosun Taekwondo Academy located in Warwick, New York and plans the Chosun Taekwondo Academy Training & Cultural Tour to Korea. Practitioners of all ranks interested in participating can reach Master Cook at chosuntkd@yahoo.com or www.chosuntkd.com.

Korean/English Translations for Taekwondo Terms

Stances

ap koobi	front stance
dwi koobi	back stance
ja choom sogi	horse stance
ap sogi	walking stance
kyorugi joombi	fighting stance
bal chagi joombi	kicking stance
bom sogi	cat stance
koa sogi	cross stance
hakdari sogi	crane stance

Kicking Techniques

ap chagi	front kick
dollyo chagi	roundhouse kick
yop chagi	side kick
dwi chagi	back kick
naeryo chagi	ax kick
bakat chagi	in to out axe kick
ahn chagi	out to in axe kick
pyojok chagi	crescent kick
miro chagi	push kick
momdollyo dwidollyo chagi	spinning hook kick
hurio chagi	hook kick
kawi chagi	scissor kick
twio chagi	jump kick
goollo chagi	hop kick
bitureo chagi	twist kick
ppodeo chagi	stretch kick
bandal chagi	half moon kick
nalla chagi	flying kick
opo chagi	falling kick
doobal dangsang chagi	double jumping kicks

Punching Techniques

momtong jiluki	middle punch
olgool jiluki	high punch
alle jiluki	low punch
bandae jiluki	reverse punch
baro jiluki	lunge punch
chi jiluki	uppercut punch
yop jiluki	side punch
dollyo jiluki	round punch
sewo jiluki	vertical punch
koondol jiluki	hook punch
dikootja jiluki	"C" punch
doo chumok jiluki	double punch

Striking Techniques

me chumok	hammer fist
doong chumok	back fist
bam chumok	middle finger fist
pyun chumok	flat fist
batang sohn chilki	palm heel strike
sohnnal chilki	knife hand strike
sohnnal doong chilki	ridge hand strike
pyun sohnkoot chilki	spear hand strike
kawi sohnkoot chilki	two finger strike
inji shonkoot chilki	single finger strike
akum sohn chilki	tiger mouth strike
gom sohn chilki	bear hand strike
sohn doong chilki	back hand strike
sohn mok chilki	ox jaw strike
palkup chilki	elbow strike
moorup chilki	knee strike
mohri chilki	head strike

Blocking Techniques

alle makki	low block
olgool makki	high block
ahn momtong makki	out/in middle block
bakat momtong makki	in/out middle block
ahn han sohnnal makki	out/in single knife hand block
bakat han sohnnal makki	in/out single knife hand block
dool sohnnal momtong makki	double knife hand block

Blocking Techniques (continued)

ghodulo makki	double closed fist block
otkolo makki	" X " block
gawi makki	scissors block
hecho makki	spread block
yop makki	side block
batang sohn makki	palm heel block
sohn mok makki	wrist block
sohnnal doong makki	ridge hand block
sohn doong makki	back hand block
pyojok chagi makki	crescent kick block
kodureo makki	double closed fist block

Basic Terminology

cha riot	attention
joombi	ready
kyung ye	bow
bal pak ko	switch stance
dwi ro dora	about face
si jak	begin
barro	return to ready
goo man	end
kibon	basics
kibon dong chak	basic movements
makki	block
jiluki	punch
chilki	strike
chagi	kick
poom-se	traditional choreographed forms
il su sik	one-step sparring
sam su sik	three-step sparring
ho sin sool	self-defense techniques
kyuk pa	breaking techniques
kyorugi	sparring
dojang	training hall
dobok	uniform
ti	belt
kukki	flag
myuk sang	meditation
shoom sha ki	deep breathing
wen	left
ohren	right

Terms of Rank

Kwan Jang Nim	Grandmaster
Sa Bum Nim	Master Instructor
Kyo Sa Nim	Instructor
Cho Kyo Nim	Assistant Instructor
Sun Ba Nim	Senior

Counting In Korean

hana	one
dool	two
set	three
net	four
dasoot	five
yasoot	six
il gop	seven
yodol	eight
ahop	nine
yol	ten

Ordinals in Korean

il	first
e	second
sam	third
sa	fourth
oh	fifth
yuk	sixth
chil	seventh
pal	eighth
gu	ninth
ship	tenth

Appendix C

Martial Arts Organizations Worldwide

Amateur Athletic Union (AAU) 1910 Hotel Plaza Blvd., Lake Buena Vista, Florida 32830, USA (407) 934-7200 www.aausports.org

International Taekwon-Do Federation (ITF) Drau Gras 3, A-1210 Vienna, Austria (43-1) 292-8467 www.itf-taekwondo.com

Korean National Tourism Organization (KNTO) Two Executive Drive, Fort Lee, NJ 07024, USA (201) 585-0909 www.kntoamerica.com

Korea Taekwondo Association (KTA) Olympic Park 88-2 Oryun-dong, Songpa-gu, Seoul, Korea (02) 420-4271 www.koreataekwondo.org

Taekwondo Times Magazine (TRI-MT Publications, Inc.) 1423 18th Street, Bettendorf, Iowa 52722, USA (563) 359-7202 www.taekwondotimes.com

The Kukkiwon (World Taekwondo Headquarters) Yuk Sam-dong, Kang Nam-ku, Seoul, 135-080, Korea 567-3201, 1058

United States Taekwondo Association (USTA) 220 East 86th Street, New York, NY 10028, USA (212) 772-8918 www.usta.info

USA Taekwondo One Olympic Park Place, Suite 104C, Colorado Springs, CO 80909, USA (719) 866-4632 www.ustu.org

World Taekwondo Federation (WTF) 5th Floor Shinmunno Bldg., 238 Shinmunno 1st-ga, Jungro-gu Seoul, Korea 11-061 (82-2) 566-2505 www.wtf.org

Yang's Martial Arts Association (YMAA) 38 Hyde Park Avenue, Boston, Massachusetts 02130, USA (617) 524-8892 www.ymaa.com

To Contact the Author:

Chosun Taekwondo Academy
62 Main Street, Warwick, NY 10990, USA
(845) 986-2288 www.chosuntkd.com or chosuntkd@yahoo.com

Glossary

Acupoints Specific locations on the body that when activated promote *Ki* flow.

Aikido The "Way of Harmonizing Energy." A Japanese system of locks and throws centered on using an opponent's negative energy against him. Founded by Morihei Ueshiba, also known as "O-Sensei."

Buddhism An Eastern philosophy turned religion focusing on self-purification and meditation. Founded by Siddhartha Gautama.

Buddhist breathing A method of breathing where the abdomen expands with the inhalation of air, and contracts with the exhalation, also called "normal breathing."

Capoeira A Brazilian martial art utilizing spinning kicks and acrobatic-like stances.

Chang Moo Kwan "Martial Training Institute", founded by Byung In Yoon

Chi See Qi

Confucianism An eastern philosophy based on social values and the role of the "superior man." Founded by the Chinese philosopher Confucius.

Cosmic mudra A traditional hand gesture shaped by the placing the back of one hand in the palm of the other while allowing the tips of the thumbs to touch.

Dan A grade of black belt ranging from one to ten.

Dantien A Chinese expression for the energy center located two inches below the navel where the internal life force resides. Also see hara and tanjun.

Do The "Way" or "Path" to enlightenment. The philosophical component of a martial art and the suffix of taekwondo as well as other martial arts.

Dobok The V-neck uniform worn by a practitioner of taekwondo.

Dojang A designated place where one comes to study the "Way," a school where the Korean martial arts are taught.

Dynamic meditation A series of exercises performed in a seated meditation intended to promote flexibility and *Ki* flow.

Free sparring A system of sparring that permits the student to utilize martial arts skills free of predetermined sequences.

Gichin Funakoshi Founder of Shotokan Karate.

Gungfu Literally translated as "good effort": a generic term for many forms of Chinese martial arts. (Also spelled "kung-fu.")

Gup A grade given to the color belt taekwondo practitioner before the attainment of the black belt.

Gwe A term for the trigrams that relate to the *I Ching*.

Hangul The Korean alphabet consisting of twenty-four characters.

Hapkido The "Way of Harmony," a Korean martial art focusing on throws, locks, hand strikes, and kicks, rich in defensive value and the cultivation of ki.

Hara A Japanese expression for the energy center located two inches below the navel where the internal life force resides. Also see *dantien* and *tanjun*.

Ho sin sool A Korean term for self-defense techniques.

Holistic approach The principle of martial arts practice that advocates uniting the mind, body, and spirit.

Hwarang An elite group of young Sillian warriors schooled in philosophy, ethics, and native martial arts.

Hwarang-do The "Way of Flowering Manhood," a set of ethical principles followed by the warriors of the Hwarang.

Hyung A traditional term for the patterns of offensive and defensive techniques practiced in a predetermined sequence by the student of taekwondo. Literally translated as "pattern." (Also see *kata, poom-se, tul*)

I Ching The ancient Chinese *Book of Changes*. Used as an oracle for guidance or forecasting future events.

Il su sik A traditional Korean term for one-step sparring, a prearranged drill where the aggressor advances one step forward while attacking prior to the defender initiating an appropriate response.

In/Yo A Japanese term for "duality of opposites." Also see *Yin/Yang, Um/Yang*.

ITF The International Taekwon-Do Federation (ITF) founded by General Choi, Hong Hi.

Jook do A Korean term for the bamboo sword.

Judo The "Compliant Way," a Japanese martial art and Olympic sport centering on throws and sweeps founded by Jigoro Kano in 1882.

Jung bong A Korean term for the fighting staff, known as a *bo* in Japanese.

Karate Literally translated as "empty hand." An Okinawan and Japanese martial art practiced in many iterations thought to be founded on fighting principles originating in China.

Kata A pattern of offensive and defensive techniques practiced in a predetermined sequence by the student of the Japanese martial arts. (Also see *hyung, poom-se, tul*)

Kendo A Japanese martial art translated as the "Way of the Sword."

Ki Korean and Japanese term for the internal life force used by martial artists to amplify technique.

Kiatsu A form of message used to balance *Ki* flow in the body.

Kihop The oral manifestation of the internal life force used by the martial artists to support technique. Also known as "spirit yell."

Kobukson A Korean battleship dubbed the "turtle boat." It was invented by Admiral Sun-Sin Yi in the 1500s.

Kong soo do "Empty Hand Way," an early name given to the Korean martial art that eventually evolved into taekwondo.

Kukkiwon The "National Gymnasium" of taekwondo located in Seoul, Korea.

Kumdo An ancient martial art and system of native Korean sword fighting.

Kwan Taekwondo school or institute. A term for the original Korean martial arts schools established during the 1940s and 1950s.

Kyuk pa Korean term for breaking techniques.

Lao gong An area at the center of the palm sensitive to *Ki* energy projection.

Makiwara A piece of canvas-covered foam mounted on a strip of wood used primarily to develop the striking areas of the hands.

Meditation A method of freeing or quieting the mind while in a seated, formal posture. Also used for visualization, *Ki* development, and relaxation.

Meridians A system of channels spanning the human body that transport *Ki*, the universal life force.

Moo Duk Kwan The "Institute of Martial Virtue", one of the original Korean martial art schools founded by Hwang Kee in 1945.

Mudra A term in Sanskrit meaning "to seal." A hand gesture used during the practice of meditation and *Ki* development exercises. Also see cosmic mudra.

Mushin The Zen concept of mind/no mind.

Muye Dobo-Tongji The "Illustrated Manual of Martial Arts" published in the 1790s; a Korean scholarly work depicting native martial art techniques.

Myuk sang A Korean term for meditation.

Oh Do Kwan The "School of My Way," one of the original Korean martial art schools founded by General Choi, Hong Hi in 1953.

Okuden A Japanese term for hidden techniques within a *kata* or *poom-se*.

Palgwe A set of eight traditional Korean taekwondo *poom-se* emphasizing low stances.

poom-se A choreographed sequence of taekwondo techniques aimed at defeating imaginary opponents attacking from various directions. (Also see *hyung, kata, tul*).

Prearranged sparring A method of sparring where students, usually clad in safety gear, are alternately assigned the role of attacker and defender.

Qi The internal life force, as expressed in Chinese, used by martial artists to support technique. (Also see *Ki*).

Qigong An ancient Chinese healing art with martial overtones based on the manipulation and balancing of *Qi*.

Sam su sik A traditional Korean term for three-step sparring, a prearranged drill where the aggressor advances three steps forward while attacking prior to the defender initiating an appropriate response

Shin shin totsu aikido "Aikido with Mind and Body Coordinated'; a form of aikido founded by Koichi Tohei.

Shinai A bamboo sword used in the practice of Kumdo and Kendo.

Shotokan Karate-Do A form of karate, translated as the "School of the Waving Pines," developed by Gichin Funakoshi.

Sieza A formal kneeling posture used during meditation practice.

Soo bahk do The "Way of the Striking Hand." A Korean martial art established by Hwang Kee upon his return to Korea from China.

Student Creed A group of tenets or moral principles recited by martial artists during the closing ritual of a class.

Subahk An ancient Korean martial art dating back to the Koguryo dynasty.

Sunbae Warriors of the Koguryo Kingdom.

Taegeuk A set of eight modern taekwondo *poom-se* emphasizing upright techniques.

Taekkyon A native Korean martial art emphasizing circular kicking techniques.

Taekwondo The "Way of Smashing with Hands and Feet." A Korean martial art and Olympic sport based on the circular principles of Chinese gungfu, coupled with the linear strikes of Japanese karate.

Tae soo do "Kick Fist Way," an early name given to the Korean martial art that would eventually evolve into *taekwondo* and *tang soo do*.

Taijiquan The "Grand Ultimate Fist." An internal Chinese martial art influenced by the principles of the *I Ching*, practiced primarily to promote health and well-being. Also known as Tai Chi Chuan.

Tang soo do The "Way of the China Hand," a Korean martial art predating *taekwondo* but active today.

Tanjun ho hup Deep breathing exercises practiced during meditation aimed at cultivating internal *Ki* energy.

Tanjun A Korean term for the energy center located two inches below the navel where the internal life force resides. Also see *dantien, hara*.

Taoism A Chinese philosophy based on the concept of non-intervention and conformity to the Tao. Founded on the teaching of Lao Tzu.

Taoist breathing A method of breathing where the abdomen contracts with the inhalation of air, and expands with the exhalation, also called "reverse breathing."

Traditional taekwondo A style of taekwondo supporting strong basic technique, self-defense tactics, *Ki* development, meditation, and *poom-se* rather than sport sparring exclusively.

Tul A traditional term for categories of offensive and defensive techniques practiced in a predetermined sequence by the student of taekwondo. Also see *hyung, kata, poom-se*.

Um/Yang Korean symbol expressing harmony between opposites. Also see: Yin/Yang, In/Yo.

USTA The United States Taekwondo Association; founded by Grand Master Richard Chun.

WTF The World Taekwondo Federation; the global governing body for WTF-style taekwondo with headquarters in Seoul, South Korea.

Yin/Yang An ancient Chinese Taoist symbol expressing harmony between opposites. Also see *Um/Yang, In/Yo*.

Zazen A form of seated Zen meditation.

Zen An Eastern philosophy and Buddhist sect based on the realization of enlightenment through meditation.

Bibliography & Sources

Choi, Hong Hi. *Encyclopedia of Taekwon-Do*. Ontario, Canada: International Taekwon-Do Federation, 1983

Chun, Rhin Moon Richard. *Taekwondo: A Korean Martial Art*. New York: Harper & Row, 1976

Chun, Rhin Moon Richard. *Taekwondo: Spirit and Practice*. Boston: YMAA Publication Center, 2003

Chun, Rhin Moon Richard. *Advancing in Taekwondo*. New York: Harper & Row, 1983

Chun, Rhin Moon Richard. *Moo Duk Kwan Taekwondo*. California: Ohara Publishing, 1983

Cook, Doug. *Taekwondo: Ancient Wisdom for the Modern Warrior*. Boston: YMAA Publication Center, 2001

Cumings, Bruce. *Korea's Place in the Sun*. New York: Norton & Co. 1997

Deshimaru, Taisen. *Zen Way to the Martial Arts*. New York: Penguin Books, 1982

Funakoshi, Gichin. *Karate-Do Kyohan*. Japan: Kodansha International, 1973

Kane, Lawrence, Wilder, Kris. *The Way of Kata: A Comprehensive Guide to Deciphering Martial Applications*. Boston: YMAA, 2005

Kauz, Herman. *The Martial Spirit*. New York: Overlook Press, 1977

Kee, Hwang. *Tang Soo Do*. New Jersey: Sang Moon Sa, 1978

Kim, Daeshik. *Taekwondo*. Korea: NANAM Publishing Co., 1991

Kim, Daeshik. *One-Step Sparring*. Korea: NANAM Publishing Co., 1985

Kim, Un Yong. *The Taekwon-do Textbook*. Korea: Oh Sung Publishers, 1995

Kimm, He Young. Taekwondo Times: *Choi Hong Hi A Taekwondo History Lesson*. Iowa: Tri-Mount Publications, Inc., 2000

Lee, Kang Seok. Taekwondo Times: *Dragon above the Clouds: An Inspirational Man Fulfills an Extraordinary Goal*. Iowa: Tri-Mount Publications, Inc., 1999

Lee, Kyu Seok. *A Guide to Taekwondo: History, Philosophy, and Training Methods*. Korea: Yeeum Publishers. 1998

LeShan, Lawrence. *How to Meditate*. New York: Bantam Books, 1974

Losik, Len. *The Kwans of Tang Soo Do*. California: SanLen Publishing, 2003

Mitchell, Richard L. *The History of Taekwondo Patterns*. Lilley Gulch Taekwondo, 1987

Morgan, Forrest E. *Living the Martial Way* New Jersey: Barricade Books, 1992

Park Yeon Hee, Park Yeon Hwan, Gerrard, Jon., *Taekwondo: The Ultimate Guide to the World's Most Popular Martial Art*. New York: Facts on File, Inc., 1986

Reed, William. *Ki: A Practical Guide for Westerners*. Japan: Japan Publications, 1986

Shaw, Scott. *The Ki Process*. Maine: Samuel Weisner, Inc., 1997

Shim, Sang Kyu. *Promise and Fulfillment in the Art of Taekwondo*. Iowa: TKD Enterprises, 1974

Shim, Sang Kyu. *The Making of a Martial Artist*. Iowa: TKD Enterprises, 1980

Suzuki, Shonryu. *Zen Mind, Beginner's Mind*. New York: Weatherhill Inc., 1970

Tedeschi, Marc. *Taekwondo*. Connecticut: Weatherhill, Inc., 2003

Tedeschi, Marc. *Essential Anatomy*. Connecticut: Weatherhill, Inc.,2001

Tokitsu, Kenji. *Ki and the Way of the Martial Arts*. Boston: Shambhala, 2003

Tohei, Koichi. *Ki In Daily Life*. Japan: Ki No Kenkyukai Headquarters, 1978

Tse, Michael. *Qigong for Health and Vitality*. New York: St. Martin's Griffen, 1995

Wei, Wu. *I-Ching Life: Living it*. California: Power Press, 1996

Yang, Jwing Ming. *Qigong for Health and Martial Arts*. Massachusetts: YMAA Publication Center, 1985

Yoo, Yushin. *Korea the Beautiful: Treasures of the Hermit Kingdom*. Los Angeles: Golden Pond Press, 1987

Yang, Jwing-Ming. *The Essence of Shaolin White Crane*. Boston: YMAA Publication Center, 1996

Index

About the Author

Master Doug Cook holds a fourth degree black belt in the Korean martial art of taekwondo and is certified in rank by the United States Taekwondo Association, and the World Taekwondo Federation (WTF). After training three times in Korea, he went on to become a six-time gold medalist in the New York State Championships, the USTA Taekwondo Invitational Championship, and the New York State Governor's Cup competitions. He holds a D3 status as a U.S. Referee and has received high honors from Korea in the form of a "Letter of Appreciation" signed by World Taekwondo Federation President, Dr. Un Yong Kim, and presented by Grandmaster

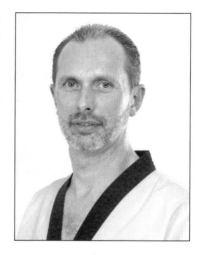

Richard Chun. In 2003, Master Cook was awarded the Medal of Special Recognition from the *Moo Duk Kwan*. In 2004, during a training camp in Korea, Master Cook received a Special Citation from the Korean government for forging a stronger relationship between the two countries through the martial arts. A six-page interview with Master Cook appeared in the May 2005 issue of Taekwondo Times magazine discussing taekwondo philosophy and his views on the role the martial arts will play in the twenty-first century.

Master Cook and his students are credited with creation of the Chosun Women's Self-Defense Course—an exciting and effective workshop geared towards women of all ages, generally offered to corporate and civic groups as a community service. Likewise, in answer to a request for training from the U.S. Army National Guard / 42nd Division, Mr. Cook developed the Chosun Military Self-Defense Course. In 2002, Master Cook was called upon to demonstrate the art of taekwondo as part of a three-man team at the annual Oriental World of Self-Defense held in New York's famed Madison Square Garden. There, he and his colleagues were cheered on by martial arts legend, Chuck Norris.

Master Cook is a traditionalist and places great emphasis on the underlying philosophical principles surrounding taekwondo. He demonstrates this belief by infusing meditation, *Ki* development exercises, strong basic skills, and attention to the classic forms, or *poom-se*, in his instructional methodology. Aside from continuing his martial arts education in New York City under the tutelage of world-renowned, ninth degree black belt Grandmaster Richard Chun, Master Cook owns and operates the Chosun Taekwondo Academy located in Warwick, New York – a school specializing in traditional taekwondo instruction and *Ki* development.

Master Cook currently shares his knowledge of taekwondo through a series of articles he has written for Taekwondo Times, Black Belt, The United States Taekwondo Journal, and other martial arts magazines. Master Cook is author of the best-selling book, *Taekwondo: Ancient Wisdom for the Modern Warrior*, published by YMAA of Boston.

Master Doug Cook can be reached through the Chosun Taekwondo Academy web site at: www.chosuntkd.com or at chosuntkd@yahoo.com. Training seminars can be arranged by contacting him at this email address.

BOOKS FROM YMAA

VIDEOS FROM YMAA

more products available from...
YMAA Publication Center, Inc. 楊氏東方文化出版中心
4354 Washington Street Roslindale, MA 02131
1-800-669-8892 • ymaa@aol.com • www.ymaa.com

VIDEOS FROM YMAA (CONTINUED)

DEFEND YOURSELF 1 — UNARMED	T010/343
DEFEND YOURSELF 2 — KNIFE	T011/351
EMEI BAGUAZHANG 1	T017/280
EMEI BAGUAZHANG 2	T018/299
EMEI BAGUAZHANG 3	T019/302
EIGHT SIMPLE QIGONG EXERCISES FOR HEALTH 2ND ED.	T005/54X
ESSENCE OF TAIJI QIGONG	T006/238
MUGAI RYU	T050/467
NORTHERN SHAOLIN SWORD — SAN CAI JIAN & ITS APPLICATIONS	T035/051
NORTHERN SHAOLIN SWORD — KUN WU JIAN & ITS APPLICATIONS	T036/06X
NORTHERN SHAOLIN SWORD — QI MEN JIAN & ITS APPLICATIONS	T037/078
QIGONG: 15 MINUTES TO HEALTH	T042/140
SCIENTIFIC FOUNDATION OF CHINESE QIGONG — LECTURE	T029/590
SHAOLIN KUNG FU BASIC TRAINING — 1	T057/0045
SHAOLIN KUNG FU BASIC TRAINING — 2	T058/0053
SHAOLIN LONG FIST KUNG FU — TWELVE TAN TUI	T043/159
SHAOLIN LONG FIST KUNG FU — LIEN BU CHUAN	T002/19X
SHAOLIN LONG FIST KUNG FU — GUNG LI CHUAN	T003/203
SHAOLIN LONG FIST KUNG FU — YI LU MEI FU & ER LU MAI FU	T014/256
SHAOLIN LONG FIST KUNG FU — SHI ZI TANG	T015/264
SHAOLIN LONG FIST KUNG FU — XIAO HU YAN	T025/604
SHAOLIN WHITE CRANE GONG FU — BASIC TRAINING 1	T046/440
SHAOLIN WHITE CRANE GONG FU — BASIC TRAINING 2	T049/459
SHAOLIN WHITE CRANE GONG FU — BASIC TRAINING 3	T074/0185
SIMPLIFIED TAI CHI CHUAN — 24 & 48	T021/329
SUN STYLE TAIJIQUAN	T022/469
TAI CHI CHUAN & APPLICATIONS — 24 & 48	T024/485
TAI CHI FIGHTING SET	T078/0363
TAIJI BALL QIGONG — 1	T054/475
TAIJI BALL QIGONG — 2	T057/483
TAIJI BALL QIGONG — 3	T062/0096
TAIJI BALL QIGONG — 4	T063/010X
TAIJI CHIN NA	T016/408
TAIJI CHIN NA IN DEPTH — 1	T070/0282
TAIJI CHIN NA IN DEPTH — 2	T071/0290
TAIJI CHIN NA IN DEPTH — 3	T072/0304
TAIJI CHIN NA IN DEPTH — 4	T073/0312
TAIJI PUSHING HANDS — 1	T055/505
TAIJI PUSHING HANDS — 2	T058/513
TAIJI PUSHING HANDS — 3	T064/0134
TAIJI PUSHING HANDS — 4	T065/0142
TAIJI SABER	T053/491
TAIJI & SHAOLIN STAFF — FUNDAMENTAL TRAINING — 1	T061/0088
TAIJI & SHAOLIN STAFF — FUNDAMENTAL TRAINING — 2	T076/0347
TAIJI SWORD, CLASSICAL YANG STYLE	T031/817
TAIJI WRESTLING — 1	T079/0371
TAIJI WRESTLING — 2	T080/038X
TAIJI YIN & YANG SYMBOL STICKING HANDS–YANG TAIJI TRAINING	T056/580
TAIJI YIN & YANG SYMBOL STICKING HANDS–YIN TAIJI TRAINING	T067/0177
TAIJIQUAN, CLASSICAL YANG STYLE	T030/752
WHITE CRANE HARD QIGONG	T026/612
WHITE CRANE SOFT QIGONG	T027/620
WILD GOOSE QIGONG	T032/949
WU STYLE TAIJIQUAN	T023/477
XINGYIQUAN — 12 ANIMAL FORM	T020/310
YANG STYLE TAI CHI CHUAN AND ITS APPLICATIONS	T001/181

DVDS FROM YMAA

ANALYSIS OF SHAOLIN CHIN NA	D0231
BAGUAZHANG 1,2, & 3 —EMEI BAGUAZHANG	D0649
CHIN NA IN DEPTH COURSES 1 — 4	D602
CHIN NA IN DEPTH COURSES 5 — 8	D610
CHIN NA IN DEPTH COURSES 9 — 12	D629
EIGHT SIMPLE QIGONG EXERCISES FOR HEALTH	D0037
THE ESSENCE OF TAIJI QIGONG	D0215
QIGONG MASSAGE—FUNDAMENTAL TECHNIQUES FOR HEALTH AND RELAXATION	D0592
SHAOLIN KUNG FU FUNDAMENTAL TRAINING 1&2	D0436
SHAOLIN LONG FIST KUNG FU — BASIC SEQUENCES	D661
SHAOLIN WHITE CRANE GONG FU BASIC TRAINING 1&2	D599
SIMPLIFIED TAI CHI CHUAN	D0630
SUNRISE TAI CHI	D0274
TAI CHI FIGHTING SET—TWO PERSON MATCHING SET	D0657
TAIJI BALL QIGONG COURSES 1&2—16 CIRCLING AND 16 ROTATING PATTERNS	D0517
TAIJI PUSHING HANDS 1&2—YANG STYLE SINGLE AND DOUBLE PUSHING HANDS	D0495
TAIJIQUAN CLASSICAL YANG STYLE	D645
TAIJI SWORD, CLASSICAL YANG STYLE	D0452
WHITE CRANE HARD & SOFT QIGONG	D637

more products available from...
YMAA Publication Center, Inc. 楊氏東方文化出版中心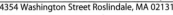

4354 Washington Street Roslindale, MA 02131
1-800-669-8892 • ymaa@aol.com • www.ymaa.com